NEW HOPE FOR PERIPHERAL NEUROPATHY

# Turn Back Your Biological Clock

*The Ultimate Guide to Better Health and Longevity*

Duncan McCollum D.C.

# Table of Contents

Author's introduction to this book

How to Fix the Cell to Get Well

Dr. Pompa's Cellular Solution Program

What is Peripheral Neuropathy? How to Reverse it?

Dr. McCollum D.C.
Dr. McClimon D.C.

7-week Cellular Healing Course

Complete Guide to Better Health
$50 Off Coupon Code

Discover Vitamin G –
the Most Powerful Vitamin on the Planet

Splurge on it! Dr. Pompa & Dr. McCollum D.C.

# Advance Praise

"I had the honor and privilege to read this wonderful book and discovered a powerful tool to help my patients on their difficult journey called healing. *Turn Back Your Biological Clock* gives the reader a nice and simplified health plan in twelve short, easy-to-read, and informative chapters. As this narrative story unfolds, the reader will discover a plan for how to start navigating their own journey of resetting their health. I have had the opportunity to work with Dr. Duncan on several occasions and appreciate his love and understanding of our patients' plight in seeking health and happiness. I find this story fun and educational. I cannot wait to share this with my community. If you want to start your healing journey or are currently confused about which way to turn, this book will lay out an easy-to-follow path for you. Thank you again, Dr. Duncan,

for helping all of us get this amazing message of healing out into the world.

— Dr. Tomas Gigena, M.D., Family Physician, True Health DPC

"Dr. McCollum is absolutely brilliant at taking difficult advanced concepts and weaving them into fun and interesting stories, making them easy for us to learn! If you want to get healthy and stay healthy for a lifetime, you will love this book!"

— Russ Rosen, D.C., CEO, The Optimal Health Coaching System

"Dr. Duncan does an incredible job helping you understand how powerful your body is. It was once thought that your genes determine your destiny. *Turn Back Your Biological Clock* makes the scientific point that you control your genes. After reading this brilliant book, you will have a complete understanding of what is interfering with your body's capability to heal, how to remove the interference, and allow your body to heal."

— Ben Azadi, Founder of Keto Kamp & Author of Keto Flex

"If there was an anti-aging guru you wanted to listen to, it would be Dr. Duncan McCollum. In his latest book, not only does he bring us the most recent research proving that we have more control over the aging process than we've been taught, but he delivers this message to us in a beautifully weaved story of hope. With his incredible depth of knowledge, his personal commitment to living the principles he teaches, and his masterful storytelling skills, Dr. McCollum is quickly becoming a leading expert in the anti-aging movement. This book will change the lens through which you view aging and give you a new insight into how you can live a life that keeps you forever young."

— Dr. Mindy Pelz, D.C., bestselling author of *The Reset Factor, Reset Factor Kitchen, The Menopause Reset*, and *Fast Like A Girl.*

# Foreword

It is my pleasure to take a moment to comment on Dr. McCollum's latest book, *Turn Back Your Biological Clock.*

This book goes far beyond any manuscript that I am aware of when it comes to this particular subject. This is not your typical anti-aging book reiterating the same old message of "eat more fruits and vegetables." As a matter of fact, some of the information will challenge your core beliefs of how we age and how we can slow down the process.

Having worked closely with Duncan over the past several years, I found him to not only look openly toward the evolving natural sciences, but also to be an early adapter, offering this information and the techniques involved to the world.

Serving as a member of the Health Centers of the Future's elite Platinum group of providers, he has significantly contributed to its expansion by bringing natural regenerative health options to his patients and clientele.

In his new book *Turn Back Your Biological Clock*, he has combined his knack for storytelling with the steps one would find necessary to reverse biological aging.

Through the process he lays out, I am confident that it is possible for the reader to get a much better understanding of what true health care is.

Our country is facing a terrible health epidemic where symptoms are traditionally covered up without addressing "upstream causes." Dr. McCollum is clear in sorting out the steps necessary to take back your own health.

I believe you will not only find the storyline entertaining, but also find many answers you've been looking for regarding your health and the well-being of yourself and those you love.

Enjoy.

In Health,

— Dr. Dan Pompa*

*Dr. Pompa is a global leader in the health and wellness industry. He is the author of the bestselling book Beyond Fasting and The Cellular Healing Diet. Dr. Pompa has spoken at organizations such as the <u>American College for Advancement of Medicine</u>, appeared on popular podcasts such as <u>The Unbeatable Mind,</u> and hosts his own podcast called <u>Cellular Healing TV</u>. He is also the principal leader and teacher of Health Centers of the Future, a group of health professionals dedicated to bringing natural regenerative therapies to those seeking optimal health and longevity.*

# Introduction

The United States is rated 47th in the world for health. Eighty million Americans are considered to suffer from multiple chronic diseases, 60% of Americans are Diabetic or pre-Diabetic, 30 million of us have been diagnosed with Thyroid disorders, we are number one in the world for obesity, we consume 50% of the world pharmaceutical drugs and yet are not even 5% of the world population. We spend 4.3 trillion dollars annually in the health industry, 70% of which is just to cover up symptoms.

Out of the fray of our failing healthcare system, a certain diagnosis has appeared, reaching epidemic proportions. Yet, according to mainstream medicine, nothing can be done about it. Peripheral Neuropathy affects nearly 2.4% of the earth's population, about 200,000,000 people globally. The percentage gets worse for those over 40 years of age. These numbers reach between 5 and 7% of that demographic. There are 25 million people in the United States who have been diagnosed with peripheral neuropathy, which would indicate that several million undiagnosed Americans are suffering with the progressive, devastating symptoms of this degenerative condition, unaware of the eventual consequences…

Peripheral neuropathy may develop abruptly due to accident or injury, but mostly begins subtilty with almost imperceivable symptoms, eventually escalating into life-altering and potentially devastating conditions. Unfortunately, traditional Western Medicine seems to believe that nothing can be done about it other than to medicate the aggressively advancing symptoms with heavy pharmaceuticals, which have terrible side effects of their own; this until more aggressive and invasive, "lifesaving" medical procedures are unavoidable.

Peripheral neuropathy is not a standalone disease, but a progressively invasive condition brought on by the gradual death of the peripheral nerves. There are many causes for this, Diabetes being the most common, but exposure to a plethora of environmental toxins, the advancing of chronic disease and often the side effects of the medical treatments of those diseases or conditions can contribute to its progression. There are many other contributors to peripheral neuropathy, but most importantly, I'm here to tell you that "something can be done about it!"

First of all, we need to stop the progression of the condition. Secondly, we need to remove the "upstream causes" which are causing the nerves to die in the first place. Even though no "magic pill" exists for this condition, you can be helped!

Several things need to happen to *"Turn Back Your Biological Clock"*. Think about your ill health as a sinking ship. First, you have to handle the emergency, bail out the boat before it completely sinks. Next, you've got to find the hole and plug it! Only then can you enjoy smooth sailing.

In this Second Edition, I will be introducing several major concepts regarding the restoration of a properly functioning and healthy body. I will be utilizing the teachings of Dr. Dan Pompa as we go over the concept of 'fasting' and the benefits and dangers of doing it correctly or not. Along with fasting, I will be discussing the Ketogenic Diet. This is how your body will learn to burn the 'other' fuel called ketones, which are derived from fats, a cleaner and healthier fuel than glucose or sugar, which has been, up to now, our body's primary fuel.

Since my first publishing, both of these subjects, fasting and ketogenic diets, have spread like wildfire over the internet, putting forth a lot of good information, misinformation, and just partial truths. This has resulted in improvements in many people's health, but also created the furthering or advancing of health issues for those either not physically fit to undertake these dietary changes, those suffering from some sort of condition which doesn't tolerate the changes or for those who do not understand the importance of such things as 'diet variation or ancient healing strategies' and go about these dietary changes 'willy-nilly' without a conceptual understanding of the health ramifications, let alone the ever-changing research.

Next, I cover the concept of detoxifying the body. There is much to be learned about this subject. This concept and practice has been around since time in memorial and has been practiced in almost all cultures, both primitive and advanced, from Native American's sweat lodges to the heated pools of the Roman and Greek empires, from potentially deadly bloodletting and mysterious rituals and even exotic snake oils.

Now, it is more important than ever to understand and utilize the safest and most effective detox protocols available if we ever wish to regain our failing health or ensure that our body is functioning at the top of its game.

But first, we must determine our end game. How do we accomplish true detoxification without stirring up the pot of stored toxins within us, which only makes us sicker?

Again, Dr. Dan Pompa stands alone with his statement 'Fix the Cell to Get Well,' and with the advances in his research and protocols, we have it nailed.

I have been extremely fortunate to be part of an exclusive group of clinicians and health coaches working closely with Dr Pompa over these past seven years. I have watched and participated in the development of these protocols and programs. When asked why he has worked so diligently in researching and developing these Core Cellular Detox protocols, Dr. Pompa earnestly replies, "For Such a Time as This. The world desperately needs what we have".

As for peripheral neuropathy, we need to curtail its progression as soon as possible. Peripheral neuropathy is the inflow of water sinking the ship of many people and must be dealt with quickly. To this end, I will introduce our Peripheral Neuropathy program, which is producing remarkable results - this in the wake of Western Medicines' failure to help this condition.

Thank you for your interest in this book, and please get it in the hands of someone you know who could benefit from it.

# Author's Note

Whatever happened to the good old days? The days that came and went? Being footloose and fancy-free?

Well, what's funny is I still feel as young as ever. I just wish my body would cooperate!

I remember hanging out at People's Park back in the early seventies, going over to Haight Asbury, and seeing shows at the Avalon Ballroom or Fillmore West. It seemed I could stay up all night, put as many unmentionable things in my body as I pleased, and still wake up refreshed (albeit at one in the afternoon).

Well, that was close to fifty years ago. The body just doesn't recover quite so easily.

One day, I was working with one of my patients, an "older lady," maybe in her late sixties. She was hard of hearing, and her body was a bit feeble. We got to talking about where she grew up. "New York," she said.

"Hum," I replied. "Were you around for Woodstock?"

"Yep," she said. "I was there."

That's when it hit me! I'm… well… my body is getting old.

I started looking at my "older" patients with a new set of eyes. These guys may have bodies that may be starting to fail, but they have amazing stories to tell.

Then I started thinking:

What happened to the rebels within us? When did we start to conform? My God, did I even say that word?

I thought we were supposed to "Turn On, Tune In, and Drop Out." Remember the famous line from the song "My Generation" by Pete Townshend of The Who, sung by Roger Daltrey, as he stuttered the words, "I hope I die before I get old / I hope I die before I get old." And don't forget Abbie Hoffman's cautionary line, "Don't trust anybody older than thirty."

Well, to any old hippies or beatniks out there who are reading this book, I guess the joke is on you! You're still alive, and so are Daltrey and Townsend at this writing!

Many of us lived our lives back then with little regard for the future, casting our fate to the wind. I guess that is how young people think. Let's call it the arrogance of youth! It may all be well and good that we did survive. We all made a living and are still here to talk about it, but at what cost?

Our quality of health in the U.S. is terrible! In fact, if you weren't aware, we are rated forty-seventh in the world for health and have been for years!

It makes one wonder: While we were all doing our thing and learning to survive, was some "faction" making a business out of keeping us sick?

- Wasn't Wonder Bread supposed to build strong bodies in twelve ways?
- Weren't Wheaties the breakfast of champions?
- Didn't Clark Kent endorse Sugar Frosted Flakes?
- And weren't PF Fliers supposed to make us run our fastest and jump our highest?

I think we've been duped!

As a historical fiction author with four published books under my belt, this educational book was written in a story format to keep it both exciting and informative. I developed some characters to represent different aspects of our current society. Today, 60% of our population is either diabetic or Prediabetic, 30 million Americans have been diagnosed with Thyroid disorders, 20 million Americans have been diagnosed with something called Peripheral Neuropathy, and 80 million Americans have been diagnosed with multiple chronic diseases. Even over 50% of our children have been diagnosed with a chronic disease. The list goes on. Something must be done about this.

In this book, I will guide you through the most current natural healthcare trends and teach you how to take charge of your health. Just like so many of my patients did, you will discover that you can change your life by taking control of your health. The processes I cover in this book have been researched and utilized by some of the greatest names in natural and restorative healthcare. I have had the privilege to know, study, and work with some of the world's top clinicians and researchers, and I am happy to share what I have learned with you.

# List of fictional characters

- **Alfred McCoy** – He narrates the story and is a typical hard-working sixty-plus-year-old who went to school, got a job, worked hard, and never thought his lifestyle would land him in a hospital bed at such an early age. He is now faced with a decision which could change his life forever.

- **Judy Jones** – Alfred and Judy met while sharing a post-op hospital room. Judy is immunocompromised and Prediabetic. She lost her husband to Diabetes five years earlier and is in need of inspiration and a glimpse of hope. A spark of love ignites as she and Alfred embark on their journey to better health and life.

- **Joey** – This is Judy's thirty-year-old son who, seeing his father's life slip away and already showing signs of diabetes and heart disease himself, turned his life around and became a health coach. I hope you enjoy how Joey walks Alfred and Judy through the steps necessary to achieve optimal health and turn back their biological clock. Throughout this story, I will be speaking and teaching through Joey, using everything I have learned over years of study and clinical practice to introduce Alfred and Judy – and you, my reader – the tools and understanding necessary to take back your health. I have walked thousands of patients through this process and have seen amazing results as the body's innate intelligence does what it does best: heal the body.

- **Alice** – Joey's older sister who is somewhat skeptical and wants to protect her mom from her little brother's crazy ideas. However, as time passes, Alice reveals some health issues of her own and stealthily begins to utilize the principles Joey is teaching.

Throughout the book, I will introduce actual people and doctors who I studied or worked with.

- **Dr. Dan Pompa** – A true leader in the cellular healing world and co-founder of the network of innovative doctors and practitioners called Health Centers of the Future, and now,

HealthCenters.com. He is the creator and developer of the Pompa Program, now the world's fastest-growing health coaching business. He continues to create unique programs based on the ever-changing understanding of the science of the human body and cellular healing.

- **Dr. Bruce Lipton Ph.D.** – A fantastic author and researcher who has taught us that the cell wall is perhaps the most intelligent and adaptable part of our body's make.

- **Dr. Jason Fung** – A renowned nephrologist and author who veered from the norm in his clinical practice and started healing his diabetic patients through diet and lifestyle.

- **Dr. Yoshinori Ohsumi** – The 2016 Nobel Prize winner in the field of medicine and physiology.

- **Dr. Valter Longo of USC** – His research on fasting and stem cell production is changing the world of healthcare.

- **Dr. Shane Morris** – A formulator and master herbalist for the supplement company Systemic Formulas.

I do cite a few other individuals to help you get a better grasp of the knowledge I am trying to give you.

I hope you enjoy the journey.

# Prologue

Alfred McCoy could be considered an average baby boomer. He grew up in the shadows of what history calls "the greatest generation." He went to school, got a job, worked hard, did what was expected, and never thought to ask too many questions regarding what life was all about. He got married, had three kids, lost his wife to cancer, and then began to fall down the rabbit hole of ill health.

By age sixty-three, he found himself in a bad way. Diabetic and asthmatic, he was alone and forlorn. Alcohol, prescription medications, and an unhealthy lifestyle while on the road as a salesman were leading Alfred to a destination unbecoming to anyone. He was slowly losing his lust for life, and a condition called peripheral neuropathy was poisoning his body and stealing his freedom.

His family rejected his communications, fed up with his self-indulging and lack of self-respect. Life's dreams were turning into nightmares, and he had little time left. Then, one day, when worse came to worst, an opportunity presented itself. Could he rise to the call?

*What is it within us that makes us decide*
*To wither or to grow tall?*
*To climb the tallest mountain or to slip and then to fall?*
*There comes a time for each of us when we have to choose*
*To cash it in or suck it up, but I'm not in your shoes*
*So take a look now deep inside and let your future be*
*Because, my friend, it's up to you to let your spirit free*
*You can decide to live or die; the choice is up to you*
*If you select the first one, then go forth with lightning speed*
*It's said two paths split in the woods, and one was seldom traveled*
*Yet therein lies the truth you seek and freedom for your taking*
*I trust in you to make your choice to let the power hidden*
*Turn on that thing that lies within and leads you to your dream*
*For youth, you'll find alive and well, just waiting for your signal*
*One if by land, Two if by sea, so let your future free*

*(in memory and appreciation of my father, who introduced me to Robert Service)*

May you find a roadmap to your dreams in the pages of this book.

With much love,
Duncan McCollum

# CHAPTER 1

# The Wake-Up Call

I was conscious for just a few minutes. The throbbing in my head blunted the sterol scent of the antiseptic room. When I finally could move my arm, I reached to find what was clogging my nose. The tubing that extended around my ears trailed off to the right and then off the bed. There was a dull burning in my right foot. When I tried to itch it with my left, there was nothing there. My right foot was gone.

Startling myself to consciousness, I forced open my eyes. I was alone. There were several machines attached to various parts of my body. I recognized what must have been a heart monitor as I focused on the dancing red line, which assured me that I was alive. The room hummed with various sounds of life-monitoring instruments.

There was a small window in the room, and as my memory began to return, I focused on a smudge spot the cleaners must have missed.

"I'll not make the fishing trip this year, I guess," I thought. I hadn't missed it in thirty-five years. One by one, the boys were just fading away. Was I the next to find my way home?

What went wrong? What happened to my dreams? Why was I here in this hospital bed at sixty-three years old, overweight, lungs failing from emphysema, diabetic, and now, due to the advancing, degenerative effects of peripheral neuropathy, minus one limb?

I did everything right – played by the book, except for the early days. Sure, I grew up in the sixties in the San Francisco Bay Area. I was there to see the riots, hung out at People's Park, and did almost every drug in the book. Well, didn't we all? But that was long ago. At that time, I guess one would call me a hippy, a dropout, or a druggie. I had no real purpose or goal except to find the next party and see where it took me.

But then again, there was the Vietnam War, the threat of nuclear power plants, and earthquakes. And, of course, hydroelectric power plants built on Northern California rivers were either heating the water too much or blocking the salmon and steelhead from returning to their happy breeding grounds. There was a lot to be mad about, and mad we were!

The greatest generation was still in power, and we were unhappy with their politics. No one knew who shot Kennedy, kids were being killed at Kent University, and no one could prove that we landed on the moon. But not only that, Joan Baez was making a stand, Timothy Leary was warping our minds, and Bob Dylan was putting it all together in his rhymes.

It's funny; I remember shopping in places like Hinks Department Store, the Co-op, Park and Shop, or Safeway and hearing all the Muzak, which played all-classical nonsense. That was a sign of the times. A time of innocence? Well, maybe a time of ignorance.

There was nothing like social media; Huntley and Brinkley reported the news while AM radio and newsprint led the parade. Big business went unchecked. Federal departments, such as the FDA, CDC, and NIH (National Institute of Health), were climbing into bed with the food and drug industry. Apparently, the FBI and CIA, along with the industrial and military complex, were experimenting with mind-altering drugs on the youths of the day. Certain powers were in the works determined to "dumb down America."

How did we get sucked into all this? We were the "dreamers;" we wanted to go back to the plow, wood-burning stoves, and even horse riding.

I was just about to dose off when the door to my room clamored open, presenting who would be my doctor making his morning rounds. He was an older, short man, about five-foot-four inches tall. His only hair presented wildly above his ears, leaving the top of his head naked. Well, actually, I misspoke – there was quite a crop exiting both ears and nostrils, as well as shadowing his eyes. His wrinkled, whitish smock spoke of the marinara sauce that apparently remained from last night's menu. And by the size of his belly, it looked as though a meal was something he rarely missed. He appeared to be rather groggy - as if he just woke up.

He looked at me without recognition, then grabbed the chart at the foot of the bed. Scratching his nose with the back of his hand, he sniffled, then pulled out a handker-chief and sneezed three times quite abruptly. I felt like telling him that if he only trimmed his nose hairs, he might solve his problem. I decided better of it.

As he rifled through my chart, which seemed to carry the balance of my life, I began to wonder who he was and why I put my life in the hands of strangers. I have always been a friendly man; my early years taught me discretion. But now, here I was, being held captive, lying flat on my back, some eighty pounds overweight and shy of my right foot.

Rasmussen – his nametag gave it away – walked over to the right side of the bed, then grabbed the sheet and flung it to the side, exposing my missing limb. Examining the dressing, we both saw the seepage, indicating the freshness of the wound.

"What do I do about the itching, Doc?" I asked in earnest.

"Don't rightly know, son. The foot's to the incinerator by now. I'll have someone come change the bandage."

With that, he dropped the chart back in the basket at the foot of the bed and exited the room. That was the last I ever saw of Rasmussen.

## My Noisy Neighbors

When I next awoke, it was to the sound of female voices engaging in quite an argument. As I opened my eyes, my orientation indicated I had moved to a different room and now had a roommate.

The curtain was pulled, but their voices were loud and clear.

"You've got to eat, Ma. You'll starve to death."

"Look at me, honey. Do I look like I'm starving? Your brother said I have enough fuel stored up in all this fat to feed New York City! And you know what, I believe him. I'm sick and tired of being sick and tired. And when I get out of this hellhole, I won't eat for a week! And that's final."

"Ma, don't be crazy. The doctor said if you don't eat, you won't get well."

"Oh, what does he know? He doesn't look very healthy himself. And besides, he wheezes like he's starving for air. I was watching a program yesterday about this thing called fasting. The guy on the TV said it was the most popular diet in America right now, and for good reason. It looked pretty interesting. It's the same thing Joey was talking about. The guy was pretty convincing. And besides, he said by not eating, you save money, don't have to go shopping, and won't have dishes to do. It sounds pretty good to me."

"Ma, that's crazy, and I'm going to talk some sense into that stupid brother of mine. Why is he always bucking the system?"

"Buck it he does, but ya' got to admit, he's the healthiest one of the bunch, and he swears by this fasting thing."

"Humph. I'm leaving, and I'm going to tell that nurse to force-feed you if need be."

With that, she stomped out of the room, leaving us to our solitude.

Hum. As I laid there taking in what I just heard, I remembered back to my childhood. Fasting. Yay. Ma would make us fast every year. What was it? Some holiday. The whole congregation did it. I liked it because that meant we could play outside longer – spring indicated that the sun stayed longer in the sky. I even remember feeling kind of good not eating. I was in pretty good shape then – quite athletic, in fact.

Then what happened?

"Clean your plate, Alfred, or you'll not get dessert!" That's what my ma said, and she was adamant about that.

Somewhere between eleven and sixteen years old, I got fat! I could never take it off. "It's just your body type, your genetics," my family reassured me. But somehow, I was never convinced. Something just wasn't right!

Like most kids growing up in the sixties and seventies, I smoked my way through high school and drank my fair share of booze. Junk food was not officially labeled as such yet, and when the first McDonald's opened up down the block, we kids were ecstatic. With McDonald's, Fenton's Ice Cream, and Dream Fluff Donuts to choose from for our late-night munchies, we had it made. Or did we?

But I kept eating and just put up with the stigma of being fat. Around the time I turned thirty, my doctor told me that I had high blood pressure and that I needed to be on medication for it. "Bummer," I thought. "Damn genetics." I was offered no other alternative.

Next, my cholesterol was identified as a killer, and some new drug was going to keep me alive.

My job kept me on the road a lot. This meant dining out, which meant a lot of fast-food meals, which could not have been healthy.

By age forty-five, I was diagnosed as pre-diabetic and prescribed other medications to keep my blood sugar level safe. A change in diet was suggested in passing but not really emphasized as too important. I was just one of those unlucky ones with bad genes. Thank God for modern medicine! I kept working.

Sara, my wife, had been a lifelong smoker and died ten years ago from lung cancer and complications of emphysema. This was sad, but no one talked about causation. Just the luck of the draw.

Our kids were all grown up and away on their own at the time. I didn't talk to them much anymore. They said I drank too much, and after Sara died, they kept their distance. I got a card or two at Christmas and my birthday, but I haven't seen the grandkids in years and didn't know a couple of the younger ones' names.

A nurse entered the room, breaking my reverie – thank God. She was pretty cheery.

"Good morning, Fred. How's the itching today?" Her name was Sally.

"Hadn't thought about it until you just mentioned it, Sally. Thanks for reminding me," I said sarcastically. "Did you find some whisky for me, dear?" She looked over her cheaters with a discerning look without comment.

Checking my vitals with the help of the attached instruments, she seemed satisfied and scribbled something on my chart.

"If you behave yourself today, Fred, you will probably go home the day after tomorrow. Have you met Miss Jones?" She asked as she pulled open the curtain.

"No," I said, "but I eavesdropped on a few conversations with her and her demanding daughter," I replied, taking in my neighbor for the first time.

"How do you do, Miss Jones? I'm Alfred McCoy."

"Pleased to meet you, Alfred. Don't mind my daughter – she has always been the bossy one. My name's Judy. By the way, what are you in for?" she asked.

"It appears they were short on right feet and confiscated mine," I replied.

"Diabetes, eh? Took my husband Mike five years ago. Advancing peripheral neuropathy, you know, kept shortening his limbs. They said it was just the luck of the draw. But my son Joey thinks otherwise. He says it could have been prevented."

"Oh, don't get yourself all worked up again, Miss Jones. That's all hogwash," Sally replied.

Just then, the door flung open, and the food cart appeared from nowhere.

"You better eat today, Miss Jones, or you will never get out of this place." Sally was stern.

"You eat it," Judy retorted. "I'm not going to touch that gruel."

"Harrumph," Sally stated as she started to pass me my plate.

"Count me out too, Sally. I'm going on a hunger strike!"

Finally, after a few more exchanges, Sally threw up her arms in disgust and stomped out!

Judy and I exchanged glances of victory and chuckled.

# CHAPTER 2

# My New Friend and Savior

"So, Judy, tell me about this fasting thing your son Joey is talking about. It sounds interesting." And so, it started.

That afternoon, Judy invited Joey over to our hospital room for an education in what he called "natural health." He was a nice-looking kid: in his early thirties, very fit and glowing. After a brief introductory conversation, I broached the subject.

"So, Joey, what's all this stuff you've been telling your mother about? What is fasting, and why would I want not to eat? Because of you, we both just went on a hunger strike. What do we do now?"

Joey paused for a minute, taking in the hospital room and his mother, then his eyes met mine. "May I call you Fred? Or would you prefer Mr. McCoy?"

"Fred is fine. Thanks for asking." It was nice to see politeness in the younger generation.

"Fasting," Joey began, "has been around since the beginning of time. Almost all ancient cultures, religions, and societies embraced and utilized it. In ancient times, the food supply varied from region to region; climate and season pretty much dictated what foods were available. Sometimes, after a harsh winter, there was no supply at all. This has been referred to as 'Starvation Spring.' Have you heard of that phrase?"

I nodded yes, saying my mother made us fast every Easter.

"Fasting has become a lost art and is one part of a much bigger subject and practice when it comes to health. Ever since World War II," Joey continued, "the availability of different foods from different countries throughout the year allowed us, especially in countries like the United States, to have any type of food from any season any time we wanted. We can get fresh melons or peaches in the dead of winter and fresh spinach, broccoli, lettuce, or avocado all year round. We have all forms of meats available at any time: dairy, grains, nuts, etc. And then there is *sugar*! Fifty years ago, the average American ate 15 pounds of sugar a year. Now, with all the sugar added to processed foods, especially restaurant foods, we consume 158 pounds of sugar a year. That's about 13 pounds a month.

"Besides all that," Joey continued, "not only has our soil been depleted of over 50% of its nutrients, but also the mass production, processing, preserving, pasteurizing, and packaging of our foods renders many of them what has been call 'dead food' with little nutrient value. More often than not, these dead foods are loaded with toxic pesticides, herbicides, additives, preservatives, and industrial byproducts."

"One more thing to discuss is the hybridization of many foods and, now, the genetic modification of so many. Wheat, for example, was dramatically modified in the 1970s. A man named Dr. Blaylock won the Nobel Prize back then for his successful modification of wheat, which allowed a yield of seven times the normal grain. At the time, this was amazing, and probably still is. His purpose was to end world hunger. In the short term, it had many advantages, but the genetic alteration of the grain created hundreds of new gluten strains that our bodies have been unable to adapt to. These glutens are hard to digest and create many bad inflammatory and allergic reactions in our digestive tracts over time. Do you remember that song 'America the Beautiful?' It has a line that says, 'Amber waves of grain.' Well, this has been replaced with 'stubby stocks of wheat.'

"We were taught to eat the worst foods possible. The famous 'food pyramid' is upside down and now basically poisoned with pesticides and herbicides. We were told that processed cereal, a glass of orange juice, and a piece of toast was the breakfast of champions! Little did we know that this deadly combination was setting up a Diabetic nation with a lowered immune response, chronic inflammation, and chronic disease!"

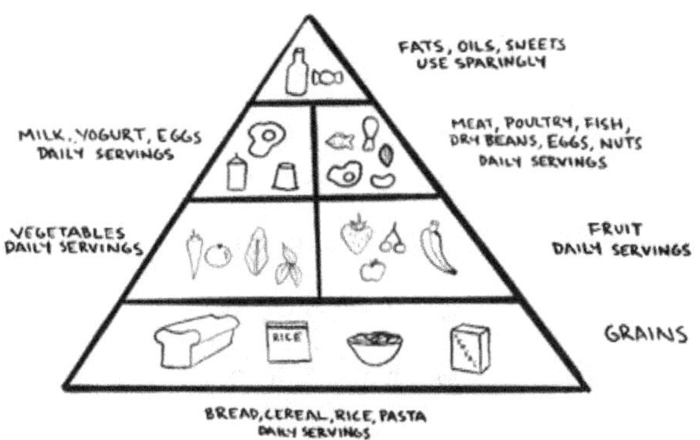


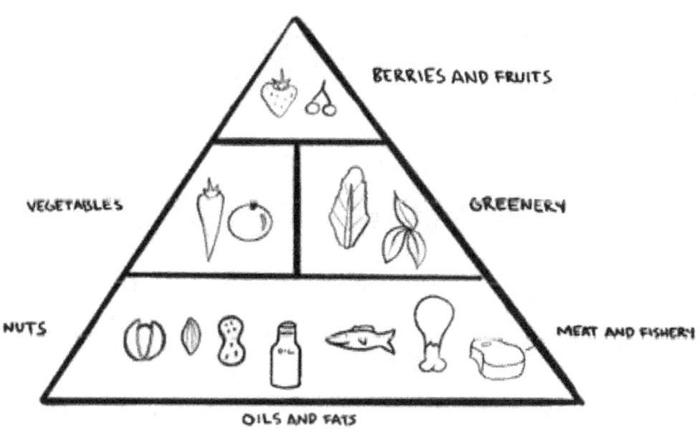


*Picture 1: The two health pyramids*

"Even today, we are told to eat six meals a day, spread nickel-injected canola oil, colored yellow, known as margarine, on our food, and clean our supersized plate, or we won't get dessert."

"So, the whole subject of commercial foods comes into play here. The first question is, what has this type of diet done to our digestive tract? Second, once the unhealthy digested foodstuffs get absorbed into our body through our bloodstream, how does it affect the different organs and their related systems, the brain, and even individual cells? You will learn how the inflammatory responses to these foods and other toxins have been devastating to the health of our populace."

"I could go on," he continued, "but at this point, I think you may get the picture. But I will say there are many more elements affecting our health and contributing to our country's failing health."

Joey took a minute and addressed me in particular. "If you are still interested, I would be more than happy to share what I learned. I want your commitment to this, though. It will be a lot of hard work and effort. As Hippocrates said, "Before you can help someone improve their health, you must make sure they are willing to give up the things that got them sick in the first place." If you don't feel up to the task, quit now and save us all some hardship. You see, my mother has no choice. I will do everything I can to help her. But your commitment is up to you. I do not wish to have someone half in the game; that would just make it too difficult for my mom."

I took a moment to appreciate the young man's integrity, then nodded and said, "Proceed. You have my commitment. I guess I really have no choice"."

Joey continued. "Let me tell you what I discovered about our country's healthcare system and the founding of 'Western medicine.'

Then, he said, "I think it is important to review the early days, the birth of Western Medicine in our country. You've surely heard of John D. Rockefeller? This man founded Standard Oil and successfully used the media, which he controlled, to push on us an article called the Flexner Report, systematically discrediting all forms of healthcare which did not fit his petrochemical model."

"He first had to rid the country of competitors such as natural, non-allopathic (not drug-oriented) healing modalities like homeopathy, naturopathy, chiropractic, botanical/ herbal medicine, and even holistic medicine. Within a few years, with the help of the media, all these other forms of healthcare were either discredited or eliminated from the United States. All medical schools that Rockefeller funded taught a curriculum representing our Western healthcare system today. How successful has this system been? I guess that depends on how you feel or profit from the state of health of our country.

"Even hemp was a threat to his plans, and since cannabis seems to have tremendous health benefits, it was also mentioned in the Flexner Report. History tells us the story here.

"It suffices to say that the Rockefeller family-run AMA and their influence over medical schools and Big Pharma shaped the direction of healthcare to where it is today.

"No doubt," Joey emphasized, "the United States has the most remarkable emergency healthcare system in the world, and there have been huge advances in modern medicine. But when it comes to covering up symptoms while allowing the diseased states to progress, rather than detecting and correcting the underlying cause, we fall short of really helping our citizens.

"Let me put it this way," Joey continued, " Does it make any sense to you that our country, which leads the free world, has the most prosperous economy, has put a man on the moon, and has provided us with tiny computers that we carry around in our pockets can't figure out how to keep our bodies healthy? Has there been any attempt to teach us about how to eat correctly or how the body has the power to heal itself? No! Well, that has to change. For us, it won't be too hard. But for the nation, it will be like trying to turn the Titanic.

"It is time for America to wake up and smell the coffee. The statistics speak for themselves. There is a better path. The words of Robert Frost in his famous poem, 'The Road Not Taken,' could hold the answers to today's health problems.

*Two roads diverged in a wood, and I —*
*I took the one less traveled by,*
*And that has made all the difference.*

"Which path will you choose?" Joey asked.

"Here is another interesting point. The American Cancer Society was founded in 1913 by ten doctors and five laypeople in New York City. It was originally called the American Society for the Control of Cancer. 'Control' – not 'cure' or 'prevention!' Today, that organization is 110 years old. Did they achieve their mission? You tell me.

"The joke or presumption is that the 'powers that be' are bent on the improbable task of 'looking for a cure' for everything when they should be focused on creating and teaching optimum health and disease prevention."

Then, he said something that hit me like a ton of bricks. He said,

"If you were in the 'healthcare' industry and you could create a drug that helped reduce someone's symptoms but never really cured anybody of anything, how long would someone need that medication? How long would they be a customer? Wow! So, the bigger question is how many drugs you could put on the market to handle the symptoms of how many diseases."

"Boom! There you have it – *'disease care or sickness care,'* the current pharmaceutical industry's purpose for existence! This is *big business.*

"Sorry," Joey added. "You asked about fasting, and I hit you with both barrels," he laughed. "Fasting is just one aspect of what you need to learn about and implement into your lives if you want to take your health into your own hands, get healthy, and get your life back."

With that, Joey stopped and looked at both of us with a look that seemed to ask, "So, what do you want to do?"

I was stunned. As I lay there in my hospital bed – obese, diabetic, asthma-ridden, and minus my right foot – I was pissed. How did I let myself fall prey to this predatory system?

I started counting the number of pharmaceuticals I was prescribed over the past thirty-odd years. I counted eighteen! All of them were designed to manage my symptoms. No one ever talked to me, other than in a passing suggestion, that there may be a way to reverse these conditions. It was implied by tacit silence that I just continued to fill the prescription until such time that the dose could be altered based on my worsening condition.

How could the government, whose job it is to protect the citizens, allow this to happen? Didn't they have agencies for this? What about the CDC and the FDA? Were they in bed with the pharmaceutical industry? Certainly not! This couldn't be!

Something started to stir inside of me – something I had not felt in a long time. I was angry, but it was a vaguely familiar type of anger - one that I hadn't felt in years, perhaps decades. I started getting memories of what my mom called "my ill-spent youth." Yes, that was it – that youthful anger when you feel like you are a small pebble on an elephant's ass. Nothing you could do could alter the path of the elephant.

Looking back now, I wonder when my generation changed. When did we decide to conform? Oh, you may think you haven't, but look again. Television, newspaper, and magazine advertisements, and now social media, have slowly brainwashed us to believe that our bodies have no ability to heal themselves whatsoever and that we are helpless when it comes to surviving without medication. Is today's media a mirror or puppet of Rockefeller's ploy of a hundred years ago? Was the media being used to control our thinking? Certainly not! Were we duped?

Einstein is often credited with that definition of crazy. It's something to the effect of, "If you keep doing the same thing and expect a different result, you are crazy." Or maybe you've got the result you are looking for.

Either way, I was done! Right then and there, I decided to take my health into my own hands. I decided to become a *"Health Rebel!"* And you know what? It felt good!

For the first time since I could remember, I felt like I could make a difference and change the world.

And so it was, a small band of health rebels, Joey, Judy, and myself, began to set a course to make a difference.

But first, we had to heal ourselves.

# The Path Less Traveled

Our first official meeting took place in a little beach house near Monterey, California. Judy invited me to drive down Friday night, and I was happy to spend the weekend as a guest at her beautiful Carmel home. It was up on a bluff overlooking Carmel's beautiful white sand beach. Judy had lived there for years. In fact, her family settled in Salinas in the 1800s. The home was wheelchair-adapted, which helped me get around while I still recovered from my surgery.

It was a beautiful Saturday morning. I spent most of the evening lying awake in my bed, listening to the ocean noisily meeting the shore, anxiously anticipating tomorrow's meeting. No one ever spent time focusing on health in my circle – just hard work, booze, and fast food.

I was up early, and as I found my way to the kitchen, I was pleased to see Judy already up, just pouring herself a fresh cup of coffee. She said good morning and gestured the coffee cup to me. I gratefully accepted. We added our cream and sugar and made our way to a little sitting nook that overlooked her garden. We visited for a while, making small talk and getting comfortable being so close together and alone.

Shortly thereafter, Joey appeared and, apparently being the cook of the family, made poached eggs for us. I noticed there was no toast and decided to be polite and not mention it. There was a small bowl of blueberries and blackberries for us, though. Following breakfast, we made our way into the den, where Joey was set up. I wondered how I would keep my stomach from growling during the class.

Joey had set up a whiteboard, a white screen, and a PowerPoint projector and had set down a stack of what looked like handouts for us to study from. Judy and I sat captivated as Joey explained what would happen for the next several weeks. At the top of the whiteboard, he wrote these words: The power that made the body can heal the body.

"So, Fred," Joey began, "before we get started, I want you to know a bit about me, my family, and our health history. This will help you understand why I am so bent on helping my mom get healthy, and I'm hoping it may help you make a decision to do whatever it takes for you to get your own life back. The Joey you see in front of you today is a completely different Joey you would have seen five years ago. You see, I grew up in a world of fast foods, alcohol, street drugs, and no real goal in life. I was easily fifty pounds overweight, and I lacked energy and drive. Then, one day, as I drove my father to his doctor's appointment, my whole perspective on my life changed. As I rolled his wheelchair and him into the sterile office, I began to get sick to my stomach. At least ten other patients were waiting to be seen, and none was there for a 'wellness check-up.' In fact, every one of them was overweight, their skin looked grayish, and they all had a sort of forlorn look in their eyes. At that moment, my life changed forever. You see, I saw myself sitting there in the near future. I was going down the same path, destined for a life of disease.

"I watched my father go from being a healthy young man teaching me to throw a curve ball to being a wheelchair-bound amputee in a little over twenty years. Nothing happened fast; it just snuck up on him. I recall hearing him tell my mom years ago that the doctor wanted him on some kind of medication for his heart. His blood pressure was too high. I remember Mom asking him if the doctor made any recommendations. 'Yes,' Dad said, 'he told me to watch my salt intake. Oh, and to stay away from fatty foods. That was about it.' Dad did neither. I recall a feeling of fear at the time and also remember thinking, *Why can't they just fix it?* Doctors were supposed to fix things, weren't they?

"And so, standing in that doctor's office, looking at all those sick people – became what was to be the turning point in my life. I started working out, determined to lose weight and get healthy. I was not going down the road of my father and all those in that doctor's office.

"I've been suffering from lower back pain since I was a kid. I am very familiar with the pain or symptom-management sickness-care system extant in this country.

"At the early age of twelve, I injured my lower back falling out of a tree on Tight Wad Hill, the famous hill that stands above the Cal Berkeley Memorial Football Stadium. I still remember my two best friends, Billy and Andy, carrying me all the way home. The doctor told my parents that I had a bad sprain and prescribed painkillers to mitigate the pain. The pain meds they prescribed never really helped the pain, and so I grew up just figuring it was normal to be in constant pain. Nobody paid attention. I would reinjure my back periodically by overdoing some physical activity or even just sitting wrong, just to be told that I was experiencing 'growing pains' and that nothing was wrong. Then, when I was entering 7$^{th}$ grade, all my friends were trying out for football. That was the first time I understood something was wrong with my back. We were all dressed up in our football uniforms, and Coach had us lifting weights, running sprints, doing pushups, etc., to get in shape, but when he asked us to do a series of several sit-ups, my lower back flared up to a point I could hardly walk. I remember seeing the look in the coach's eye; it was like he just looked through me like I was nothing, and he just didn't see me anymore. After that, I often felt anxiety, grief, or insecurity at not being able to do the physical things my friends could do without suffering flare-ups of my severe lower back pain.

Looking at it now, not being able to participate in that group of friends was kind of a turning point for me. I eventually found a new group of friends, but only these guys hung out in the park. Soon, I turned to street drugs and alcohol in an attempt to relieve my pain. These only added to my problem, and in fact, the chronic abuse of the combination of them almost killed me.

The drugs had other drastic effects on me. I was diagnosed with dyslexia in first grade and had never really learned to read. One day in third grade, we were in circle time, which meant we all took turns reading out loud. I was scared to death. To my right sat John; he was completely blind, yet when it came time for him to read, he read beautifully with his fingers, "See spot run." When my turn came, I stumbled, looking at the characters on the page, wishing I was anywhere but there. I could not read a thing. The worst part was the embarrassment, especially because the girl I liked was sitting beside me. Over the years, the drugs I consumed only worsened this condition.

Drugs and alcohol became a big part of my life, impairing not only my reading ability but often my judgment. Foolishly, I continued to work out anyway, not comprehending what had happened to my back. Then, one day, after a bout at the gym, I woke up in severe pain and couldn't get out of bed. Finally, my doctor ordered an MRI and told me I had ruptured a disk and needed immediate surgery.

My father had just passed away, and all I could think about were his operations: first one leg, then a year later the other. His doctor called his condition 'Peripheral Neuropathy', some fancy word that meant the nerves in his legs and feet were dying. He said that the diabetes was causing his red blood cells to become sticky (sticky because of the exorbitant amount of sugar in his bloodstream) and that they were clogging the tiny blood vessels called capillaries at the tips of his toes. This was cutting off the oxygen supply to his feet. He explained that oxygen was necessary not only for the cells to survive but also for the nerves to have a constant blood and oxygen supply. The drugs that they gave him never solved this problem, so the wounds never healed correctly, and the blood poisoning eventually got him.

So when my surgeon ensured me that the surgery was safe – that he had performed dozens of low back operations and had a reasonable success rate – I started wondering what 'success' really meant. After all, they successfully removed my dad's left foot – that was what they intended. What they didn't take into account was the blood poisoning that developed from the wound. It killed him three weeks after the "successful" surgery.

"I started researching low back surgeries and found these statistics: 30% of the time, the pain resolved; 30% of the time, it remained the same; and 30% of the time, it got worse. There was a 10% variable. One article I found from the NIH National Institute of Health stated that in 2004, the cost of lower back surgery in the U.S. exceeded $16 billion. It went on to mention that 10-46% of the surgeries were failures. So, in my eyes, almost $8 billion was spent on surgeries that didn't work! When I asked the doctor about this, he confirmed there was no guarantee. In my mind, I figured I had a 60 to 70% chance of being the same or even worse. Therefore, surgery was not an option for me. I had to find a better way.

"I still could not stand or hold myself up and remained flat on my back. No painkillers touched the pain. My friends had to help me with bed pans; if I could eat anything, they spoon-fed me. I have to tell you, I almost gave up. I was seriously thinking of ending it all. I watched my father suffer so much, and I could not see myself going down that road.

"Then, one day, two friends came in and said they were going to take me to a chiropractor. '*What?*' I shouted in protest, which shot a bolt of lightning-like pain down my right leg."

'No way. I am not going,' I proclaimed as I recovered from my agony.

'Sorry,' they said, 'you have no say in the matter.'

"Then, they picked up an old green couch I had in the living room, put it in the back of my own pickup, lifted me up, put me on the couch, and drove me to the chiropractor's office."

"I remember them carrying me into the doctor's office. I was scared to death. But then, my eyes landed on the beautiful receptionist. Her name was Patty. She was from the Midwest, and her lovely pale skin, perfect complexion, and angelic mannerisms reminded me of Snow White. She instantly calmed my nerves. She welcomed me into her office and even filled out the paperwork for me. I remember her putting her hand on mine, calmly looking into my eyes, and saying, 'You're safe here. The doctor will help you.' Somehow, I believed her or wanted to. I wanted to live."

"What happened next was nothing short of miraculous. Dr. Duncan McCollum came to greet me and, seeing that I could not walk, asked my two friends to assist him in carrying me to the exam room. He questioned me about my back, my general health, my family history, etc. I listened to his sincerity and began to have hope. This man really seemed to care. Next, he said he needed an x-ray, explaining that the MRI being taken while I was lying down would not give him the information he needed. Seeing again that I could not walk, let alone stand, he asked my two friends if they would be willing to hold me up in front of the X-ray machine. They agreed.

"I remember lying on Dr. McCollum's chiropractic table thinking that my life was over when he finally came out of the darkroom and put my X-ray up on the view box. Then, something amazing happened. He pointed to a spot on the X-ray and said, 'When did you break your back?'

"I felt like I was hit with a ton of bricks! I could see the bone in my lower back was misshaped; it looked crushed. That was when I told Dr. McCollum about the fall from the tree when I was just twelve years old. Now I was twenty, and in all the years of back pain, no one had ever seen fit to take an x-ray! Somehow, I felt betrayed; anyone could have seen the broken vertebra, but nobody bothered to take an X-ray. I guess I was lucky they did not discover this when I was younger because they may have done surgery earlier, and who knows where I'd be now?!

"Dr. McCollum said he was very concerned that I hadn't had a bowel movement in a week and pointed to my squished vertebra, saying that the nerve that exited the spine at that level controlled the large intestine. He said he could help but wanted me to agree that if he couldn't, he wanted me to go to the emergency room and that surgery may be my only option. He talked to my two friends and got their agreement that they would see to it that I got to the hospital if he couldn't get the pressure off my nerves.

"What he did next was amazing. He helped me lay on my right side, putting me into some weird position, and then gave me my first chiropractic adjustment ever. *Wow* – there was a big pop in my back, which made my heart race and my body sweat, but what was amazing was that I felt immediate relief. I was still in pain, but I was able to stand on my own two feet and, for the first time in three weeks, walk by myself.

And that was just the beginning. Dr. McCollum continued to adjust my back and also started working with me to lose weight. He said that I was Prediabetic and that I better take my health seriously, or I'd follow in the footsteps of my father.

"That did it."

"You see, Fred, that is why I am here today. I worked on learning about health these last five years, and I feel better now than I have since I was a kid."

"So, Fred," Joey announced, "Here is the million-dollar question: If it is possible to recover your health while at the same time turn back your biological clock, is now a time in your life that you will do whatever it takes to make this happen?

"If your answer is yes, then for the next several weeks, we will not only be discussing how to do this, but will also start implementing the process of turning back your biological clocks. If you agree, that process starts right now!"

As I voiced my agreement, Joey passed out a couple of sheets of paper. One was titled "Keto-Friendly Shopping List," and the other was "Goals." He said that we should take a minute to peruse the food list and that we would go over the goals section after lunch.

Right about then, Judy's daughter showed toting a tray of coffee and a box of doughnuts that looked like it came from the corner gas station! Apparently, she'd heard about the meeting from her mom and wanted to make sure we were not being misled by her "system-bucking" little brother, Joey!

Alice was introduced to me officially by Joey, then with the caveat of, "What the hell are you doing here? And what the hell do you have in that box?" I could tell there was no love lost between the two.

"Mom invited me. She thought I'd be interested. Oh, this box?" she said, indicating the box in her hand. "Just some snacks. I stopped by Dream Fluff Donuts on my way down. Mom loves the jelly-filled!"

Now, that got my attention. I grew up in Berkeley, and Dream Fluff was just down the block from where I lived. In fact, I say much of my acquired tonnage as a young lad could be attributed to the famous donut holes mom would bring home frequently. Seeing the white box labeled Dream Fluff was almost a deal breaker – that was until Joey interrupted.

"Damn it, Alice, I think you are trying to kill her! Get those disgusting things out of the house now!"

The conversation ensued was fairly explosive and filled with expletives I'd rather not repeat. At any rate, they finally calmed down with a bit of help from Judy's long-practiced mediation skills.

The final verdict was that Alice could stay so long as she didn't interrupt the meeting. The donuts? They went to the kitchen. The coffee was allowed, but either black or with whole whipping cream – no sweetener, yuck.

What amazed me was that just a couple of weeks ago, I would not have thought twice about helping myself to two or three donuts. Even then, I was somewhat tempted.

Besides that, during the confrontation, I secretly reviewed the list of approved foods Joey passed out. Sadly enough, donuts were not to be found!

After things calmed down, Joey started again, opening up the PowerPoint, which projected on the white screen.

Joey looked at us for a moment as if in reflection, then taking a big breath and letting it out, he began.

"Look, I am glad you are here, Fred. Please excuse my sister for her interruption and our emotional outbreak. As siblings, we've been at it for years. I hope you can take in the information I will go over these next several weeks and use it to change your health without more misguided disturbances by my family."

Clearing his throat as he looked quizzically at his sister, he said, "Now, if you don't mind, Alice, I am going to continue my class."

As all eyes turned to Alice, she acquiesced – her body language suggested she would remain quiet.

Looking right at me, he said, "I really need to know your commitment level. I will ask you throughout the program if you are still in. I'm here for my mom, but I am willing to have you tag along. What are your thoughts, Fred?"

I was amazed. How could the average American barely know anything about what he had just covered? We were all so busy raising families, trying to make ends meet, keeping up with the Joneses… wait a minute, these are the Joneses. I laughed out loud. Judy, Alice, and Joey Jones – how ironic.

"I'm in, Joey," I said. "Besides, what options do I have? I looked down the path I'd been traveling on, and I didn't like what I saw. I feel like this is exactly where I need to be. This is very interesting and exciting; quite honestly, this is the first thing I've been excited about in years" (Except your mother, I wanted to say, but thought better of it). You lead the way, my friend. I'll follow the path less traveled. Besides that peripheral neuropathy thing is what took my right foot; I remember my doctor warning about the symptoms I was having a few years earlier; I just didn't pay attention. I never thought anything like this could ever happen to me. Surely, I don't want to lose my left foot; one's enough! I'm already feeling an increase in the numbness and tingling in it, and the bed sheet bothers my foot at night. That is how it started with my right foot, and I'm scared about my left."

"Okay," Joey replied. "I completely understand, but here's the deal. Before you say yes, I want you to know that each week for the next seven weeks, we will be meeting to go over key information that will lead you through what's called a Cellular Healing Lifestyle Program. I propose that we meet here at my mom's house on the weekends to review the previous week's progress and to study and prepare for the next week's lesson. Are you up for that?"

Whoa. I had not really committed to much in the last several years. I felt a bit of fear well up inside of me. I was wondering if I could do it. Could I make the commitment? Something inside of me told me that this was the one, perhaps last, chance that I would have. Who else would be willing to do this for me... and with me? I sat deep in thought, again contemplating what Joey said, unaware of the time passing. As I precipitously came out of my state of introspection, I looked over to Judy. She was sitting quietly, looking into my eyes. She must have sensed my embarrassment and internal struggle, and her glance seemed to tell me, 'Yes, you can do it.' There was more to it, though; I felt needed. I felt we were in this together. 'Please, come on this journey with me.' Her eyes seemed to be telling me.

I suddenly felt like that character, Clark Kent, who had just walked into a phone booth and tore off his 1950s-style suit, only to emerge as *Superman*. "Faster than a speedy bullet, more powerful than a locomotive, and able to leap tall buildings at a single bound."

Not only was I ready for the task, but I was also willing and felt as capable as I ever had. I was excited and, for a moment, felt like a kid again. This was going to be a fun and rewarding adventure. Besides that, I had Judy to do it with!

"Let's get started, Joey," I almost demanded. "I'm ready to go. I'll stick with it and see it through to the end. You have my word on that, and besides," I said as I looked over to Judy's beautiful smile beaming at me, "I wouldn't want to let your mom go through this alone. I think she needs my moral support."

With that, we all laughed, breaking the tension of the moment and clearing the way to our new beginning.

"Fantastic," Joey remarked. "Let's get going!"

"I want you to know you are wise to do this now. I remember the first time my dad's doctor mentioned the nerve damage in his feet. That's the first time I heard of peripheral neuropathy. I started researching it and discovered that over 25 million Americans have been diagnosed with it. What's scary is that probably twice that number are developing peripheral neuropathy with no idea that they are. I had no real understanding of how the bloodstream supplied oxygen to the nerves. It made sense to me that the cells in our body needed oxygen to survive. As diabetes progressed, the sticky red blood cells could get stuck in the small arteries and clog them. But it was news to me that there was what is called a protective 'myelin sheath' around our nerves, even the tiniest of them at the tips of our toes. Apparently, this 'myelin sheath' nourishes and protects these nerves, and without a good supply of oxygen to them, not only does the sheath break down, but with it, so does the nerve die. This then leads to the destruction of the surrounding muscle and skin tissue, and the bones begin to decay. The good news is that the research shows that the peripheral nervous system (all the nerves outside of the spine) will continue to grow for all of our lives as long as there is an oxygen supply. Of course, it is also imperative to provide nutrients while, at the same time, removing the toxic load damaging the delicate nerves.

*Picture 2*

*Scan the QR code to learn about Peripheral Neuropathy*

# PERCENT PERIPHERAL NEUROPATHY NERVE LOSS

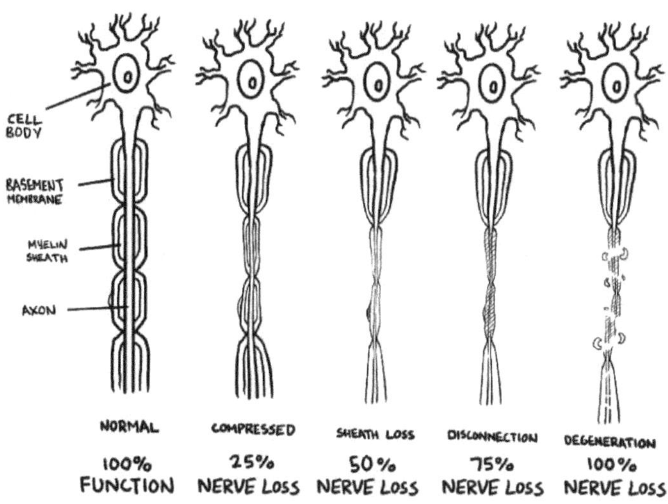



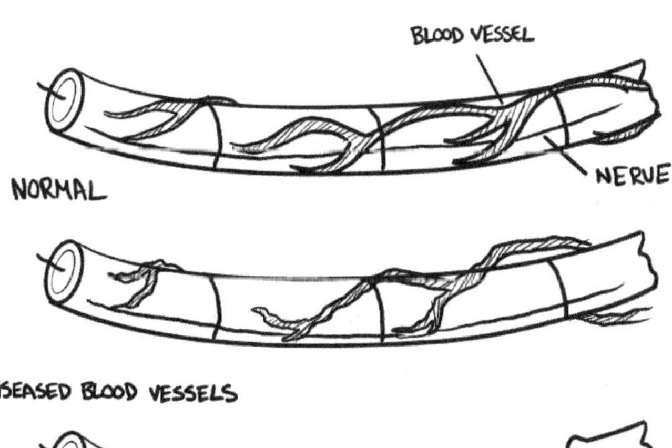



*Picture 3*

During the next seven weeks, we will be going over how to not only stop further nerve death, but also find out what is causing the nerves to die and, better yet, what to do about it. Moreover, we will be learning about chronic inflammation, its prevalence, what causes it, and how it is the leading cause of all chronic diseases, be it what is called autoimmune, where your body is fighting itself, genetic or toxin-induced.

"So, if you're ready, let's get started."

## Cellular Healing Lifestyle

"Okay," Joey said, "Now I'm going to explain what the seven-week Cellular Healing Diet is all about. In these seven weeks, we will begin to transform the way your body burns fuel, what fuel it burns, and when. This allows your body to heal the damage done to your digestive system and begin the reduction of inflammation in your body.

"We will help your body begin to break down old (senile or senescent, often coined Zombie cells) and rebuild your body with an increased production of your own stem cells. The cool thing is that you should start to feel better in a few weeks, if not a few days.

There are a few terms and concepts that I want to review with you now, but rest assured that we will go over them in more detail as time goes on.

**Stem Cells**

"First, let's look at what stem cells are and understand that they are newly created cells that can become any of the 200 different types of cells in your body. I'm sure you have heard the term Stem Cells by now, but not everyone really grasps what they are. Stem cells are the basic cells in your body. When an egg and sperm come together, I'm not going to discuss how or when that happens," this got a chuckle out of both Judy and myself, "and create the initial stem cell containing all 23 pairs of genes, the DNA coding and every aspect of what our bodies will become, the miracle of life begins. This initial stem cell divides and divides until today. I'm looking at about 75 trillion cells in each of you, each cell doing 60 million functions a minute, all controlled by the brain. Well, your body continues to make these single stem cells throughout your life, and since they contain all the DNA, these stem cells can become any type of organ, cell, or tissue in our body.

These stem cells lay dormant in the bones of your body. They just haven't 'differentiated' or decided what type of cell or tissue to become yet. They are just awaiting 'assignment' once they are called to a location." Joey went on to explain, "The older you get, the fewer stem cells you have and the slower they are to respond to the demands of your body for repair. But the good news is that you can induce and increase the production of these stem cells through fasting and other means we will discuss as we go along."

## Zombie Cells

"Senescent or Zombie Cells, by the way, are cells in your body that have either outlived their life expectancy and now are either a burden to your health and wellbeing or have mutated into what is basically an enemy to your health, aka cancer cells or otherwise damaged cells and tissues."

## Autophagy

"I have been studying this very cool process called 'autophagy." Auto means "self," and "-phagy" means "to eat." So together, the term means 'to eat thy self".

Your body can break down old and damaged cells through this process, autophagy. Autophagy is always happening, but you can speed it up, causing the body to destroy the broken-down cells and rebuild new cells out of the recycled cellular waste," Joey continued. The Nobel Prize winner Dr. Yoshinori Ohsumi won his award in 2016 partly for discovering that your body breaks down your cells rapidly after a three-day fast. This is important because those old, tired, dysfunctional, or mutated cells cause disease. So, by fasting, we are inducing a deep cleaning of the body's older and spent cells.

## Apoptosis

Apoptosis is another term we should become familiar with. This means 'programmed cell death'. Believe it or not, every cell in your body has an expected cellular life cycle or life span. We can call it a cellular 'cycle of life.'

The cell's life begins, ages, and then dies. Just like we do as an organism, only there are trillions, if not quadrillions, of sort cellular life cycles that occur in our body during our life. Crazy, isn't it?

An important point about apoptosis is the expected lifetime of the cell. One thing the physical, chemical, and emotional stressors have done is mess with the apoptosis programming. In other words, the cells aren't dying like they are supposed to; they either die sooner, mutate into something disastrous, or just become zombie cells, sucking up your valuable energy and other life-sustaining resources. In any case, it is not a good scenario. In a healthy body, apoptosis occurs appropriately. Then, the material the cell is made of is either burned for energy, recycled to make a replacement cell, or eliminated from the body. More on this later.

"Another scientist named Dr. Valter Longo from USC had discovered that stem cell production was at its highest after a three-day water fast. This is another reason for you to learn to fast, so your body can create many more stem cells that replace your old, tired, sick, or worn-out, senescent, zombie cells with brand new ones."

"So," Joey said, "fasting or not eating for a set period will not only help you break down old cells more rapidly but also prompt your body to replace them with new, young, healthy cells. This is cool." Then he said, "Also, there are these things called *telomeres*, found at the end of your DNA strands. These telomeres are kind of like those horsetails that you find down by a pond. You know, the one you pull apart section by section until there is nothing left. Well, these telomeres are kind of like those. Each time a cell in your body divides, the telomere gets a section shorter. Once the telomere is gone or there are no longer any sections to divide off, the cell will no longer replicate and either dies or becomes senescent, a.k.a. senile or zombiesque. These old, spent cells are unhealthy and can mutate and cause disease. So you see, you want to break down and recycle these old cells as rapidly as possible; by doing so, your body can actually get biologically younger.

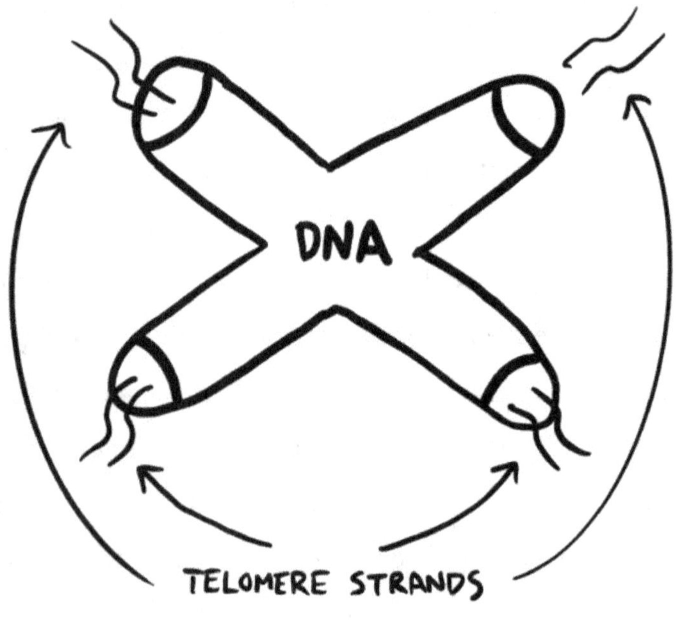


*Picture 4: Telomeres*

"You see," Joey continued, "research proved that by fasting correctly, your telomeres can lengthen or become longer. Fasting, along with other practices we will go over, can reverse or turn back your biological clock! Isn't that way cool?"

I was excited and ready to go.

Joey said that we could order a kit to get our biological age tested. There was a site offering them called teloyears.com, and it cost about $100 to get them tested. We all agreed that it would be fun to do, so on the next break, Alice went ahead and got them ordered for us. Why not, right?

## 7-Week Plan

*Scan the QR code to register for the 7-week course*

Now Joey was ready to give us the plan.

"In this first week, you will make great strides. All three of you are in the beginning phases of converting your body into fat- or ketone-burners. In this first week, our goal is to get off of what has been termed the "Blood Sugar Rollercoaster." You see, rather than explain it, I just want us to get started and then explain the process as we go. As you learn to implement more of a ketogenic diet and life-style, you will start to feel less irritable, calmer, and more stable mood-wise. This is because your body will begin to be able to recognize and utilize your hormones. This is called hormone optimization. We will talk much more about it later.

"Starting today, you will learn to keep track of the amounts of each food type you consume," Joey continued. "A ketogenic diet done right, I must state, is high in healthy fats and oils, moderate in protein, and lower in car-bohydrates. This combination will slowly convert your body into an efficient fat burner. This will lay down the foundation and prepare your body to lose the weight you've been accumulating for years or burn the old toxic fat cells in your body, replacing them with new, healthier cells. Basically, your diet will consist of 60% fats, 50 net grams of carbs, and low to moderate amounts of protein.

"Now, I want to introduce to you what's known as the 2-2-2-2 Rule. This is where we consume six tablespoons of fat or healthy oils a day and two teaspoons of sea salt, not to be confused with table salt, which is basically sodium chloride but something like Himalayan sea salt. This is loaded with a wide array of the minerals needed for a healthy body."

Joey could see the shock in my eyes. My doctors always told me that I should avoid salt, that fats were bad, and that I should eat small portions of carbohydrates daily. This was a completely different story. I mentioned as much.

"I totally understand," Joey said. Then he asked, "How long have you been following those directions? And did your health get any better?"

"For years," I said, "And no, my health got worse. Look, I'm even minus a foot to boot – no pun intended."

"Right," Joey said. "My dad listened to the same advice, and look where it got him.

I had to agree.

"Okay," Joey said, "let's go over healthy oils and fats. So, we want to consume six tablespoons of any of these healthy oils daily: olive oil, coconut oil, ghee, avocado oil, grass-fed butter, whipped cream, or *MCT oil (medium chain triglycerides)*. By the way, organic is a must!"

*Scan the QR code to watch 'Eating Healthy Oils to Support Your Cellular Health'*

Joey went on to explain what an MCT was: coconut oil with one fatty acid, lauric acid, removed. That is the one that made coconut oil hard at room temperature. He said that MCT oil could cross right into the cell and into the *mitochondria,* which he explained to be the powerplant or carburetor of the cell. He said that consuming these oils would not only get my body into ketosis, which means burning fat instead of sugar as the primary fuel faster, but would also keep me feeling full and energized as my body became accustomed to a low-carb diet.

Joey passed out another chart and told us he wanted us to start tracking our daily oil consumption for the next week. He also wanted us to mark down how many times we put any foodstuff in our mouths.

"Today, as we start Week 1 of the Seven-Week Cellular Healing Lifestyle course, I will be giving you everything you need to understand so that you can take control of your health. The course was developed by Dr. Daniel Pompa, one of the world's foremost leaders in cellular healing. It is exactly what I followed to turn myself around. You will learn a lot about how your body works so you can make good dietary decisions now and in the future.

"Each week, we will learn steps toward implementing dietary and lifestyle changes designed to walk us back up the path to freedom. I say freedom because, looking at both of you, I see two beautiful souls trapped in aging and ailing bodies waiting for the other foot to drop... oops." Joey looked at me and said, "Sorry, Fred, maybe that wasn't the best metaphor."

I laughed and told him it was a completely accurate and appropriate statement, to worry not and to carry on.

He passed out a couple of lists, then said, "Starting today, we are going to eat only foods off of this list. These will help get us off of the already mentioned blood sugar rollercoaster that is killing our fellow citizens.

"Here are some of the rewards you will reap by implementing the ketogenic diet:

- Weight loss
- Mental clarity
- Calmness
- Reduction of food craving
- More energy
- Stronger immune system
- Reduction of brain fog
- Improved digestive function
- Hormone Optimization
- And maybe most important of all, FREEDOM!

"Well, tied with first place is hormone optimization. Hormones control your body by responding to information sent from the hypothalamus, the master gland of the endocrine system. When your body is inflamed, hormones have a hard time relaying signals to or acting on the cell, which is their sole duty, and your body struggles to function correctly.

"So, now I want to go over how eating a high-fat, moderate-protein, and low-carb diet will not only make your body a better fat burner, which it looks like all three of you need – but also help rebuild your immune system, repair your digestive system, and start turning back your biological clock. That's something all of you could use, right?"

Joey purposely looked at his sister, who let out a guttural "Harrumph!"

Again, that drew laughter from the group.

Getting our attention again, Joey said, "For this first week, we will be concentrating on eating what is termed a Keto-Friendly Diet. First, this will consist of no simple carbs – no grains, breads, sugars, potatoes, etc. Secondly, we will focus on eating 'complex carbs' (live vegetables). Thirdly, healthy unprocessed meats, and fourthly, healthy oils and fats. All of this will be organically grown or organically fed in the case of meats, and you will consume no GMO foods."

There was a knock on the door. As we looked up, Joey announced, "In fact, perfect timing. It's time for lunch. Today's menu is freshly baked Monterey Bay sea bass and butter lettuce salad with plenty of avocado oil, smothered in a blue cheese sauce, and topped with toasted pecans, blueberries, fresh basil, and ground pepper. After lunch, we can spend some time answering your questions and reviewing your health goals. Thank you very much for allowing me to help you. I must say, it is encouraging to see you all so engaged!" With that, I noticed Alice moving uncomfortably in her seat.

Lunch was served in a small dining room that overlooked a beautiful garden shaded by coastal oaks. I recognized the rhododendrons, azaleas, and jasmines intermingled with cyclamen and primrose. I felt a bit nostalgic as I recalled a time long ago when my wife and I spent time in our garden. But that was long ago and far away. I mentioned to Judy that I used to love gardening in another lifetime. She touched my hand and offered me to help her pull weeds anytime. There was a chuckle from around the table. Alice confirmed her mom made her the same offer many times and tried to explain to me how fun it could be. Somehow, I felt like Tom Sawyer was talking me into whitewashing a fence somewhere. I mentioned as much, which got another chuckle.

As we enjoyed the amazing meal Joey provided, I perused the shopping list he passed out, as well as a list of approved foods. It looked pretty doable, but no bread? This is going to be tough. I loved bread! Thankfully, the meal was fantastic, and I thought, "If all the food is this good, I can get used to this." But I was sad to see that donuts were not on the approved list.

I must say, I could get used to this! The food was delicious, and the conversation was easy. I felt comfortable and somehow felt a happiness arise in me that I had not felt in years.

Following an incredible lunch, Joey directed us back to our studies and started by asking if there were any questions.

I brought up the concept of not eating bread and how difficult that might be. I could feel a heavy weight lift as I did so – no doubt both Judy and Alice had similar thoughts.

"This is a common concern," Joey remarked. "I had the same feeling and concern, but after the first day or two, I didn't really miss it. You'll see. I'm sure it will go that way with you, too.

"Now," Joey said, "another assignment for the week is to stay away from snacks. Studies show that the average American puts foodstuff in their mouth up to seventeen times a day. This could be a sip of soda, an apple, gum, a candy bar, beer, or wine. Anything other than water will spike your own body's insulin level as these foods turn to sugar or glucose in the body. I'll explain more about this as we go along, but for now, just go with me here. You will understand more about it later."

"Gum?" I inquired. "Why is that?"

"That's a fair question, Fred," Joey remarked. "You see, the flavor of the gum, whether sugar-free or not, has a sweetness to it. This sweetness can trigger the brain to think you are consuming something that would burn as glucose. This, again, can trigger the release of insulin by the pancreas. One of our goals is to reduce your body's dependency on glucose-producing foods. You will understand more as we go. Trust me, and you will thank me later.

"Now that you've consumed your first keto-friendly meal, I want you to turn to the page titled, 'Keto Friendly Shopping List.' Take a minute to read down the list to familiarize yourself with your new favorite foods."

Alice looked up and announced, "There are no donuts listed here!"

I mentioned that I noticed the same thing, which drew a big laugh from the room. I was beginning to like her.

Next, Joey directed us to the "Your Health Goals" page and asked us to take a minute or two and write down what we would like to see health-wise in six months.

"Pretend you have a magic wand and forget everything you 'think' can't happen. Just get creative!"

"Great. Now, everyone, open the camera on your phone and hand it to me." When we all looked a bit confused, Joey said, "I am going to take a picture of you, full body, and a close-up of your face. Don't worry, I won't post it on Facebook, TikTok, or Instagram. But you will be delighted when we compare photos in a few weeks."

After our photoshoot, Joey said we would calculate our body mass index next.

"Your body mass index – or BMI for short – can be measured with a fairly simple math equation," he explained. "It measures our body fat based on height and weight. It's easy to calculate and helps us gauge our general health risks and disease susceptibility. Everybody, pull out your cell phones, and let's do it together right now!" Joey suggested.

We all scrambled for our phones as Joey wrote the equation on the whiteboard.

## Body Mass Index Calculator

Take your body weight in pounds, then multiply that by 703. Now, divide that number by your height in square inches.

Joey's numbers: 703 times 170 pounds divided by 70 inches squared (70 x 70).

119,510 divided by 4900 = a BMI of 24.4

BMI Categories:

- Underweight = < 18.5
- Normal weight = 18.5 – 24.9
- Overweight = 25-29.9
- Obesity = BMI of 30 or over

I did my calculation and measured way over the 30 mark. I didn't ask Judy or Alice what theirs were, knowing I was clearly the winner.

"Don't despair," Joey said encouragingly. "This is a starting point; it's going to change. You'll see.

"Imagine driving a Volkswagen up a steep hill," Joey offered. "Also, imagine that you have the truck filled with old library books and that the motor was a quart low of oil. How easily do you think that bug would get up the hill? Not very easily. Especially if you tried to floor it on a hot summer day! It would probably blow up, right?"

"Now, imagine a well-tuned Ferrari with nothing in the trunk. It doesn't matter what time of year it is or anything. If you put the pedal to the metal on that thing, it would fly up the hill."

"Having a BMI over 25 and especially over 30 from the math equation we just solved indicates that not only are you carrying too much body fat, but that you also have inflammation in your body and likely a weak digestive system. You are probably suffering from one or more chronic disease processes at any stage of development. This means your body is like that old Volkswagen struggling to get up and over the mountain."

"Over the next few months, we are going to overhaul your health and get you burning more of the cleaner fuel and in the right mounts, these being ketones rather than chugging along predominantly on the cheaper, dirty-burning fuel known as glucose, or sugar."

## Chronic Inflammation

Clicking the remote to the projector, Joey revealed a picture of the cover of *Time Magazine*. On it was a surreal picture of a human body. The title was "Inflammation: The Silent Killer."

"In order to reverse the effects of chronic inflammation on your body and its path to chronic disease, we need first to understand where inflammation comes from. Almost every magazine and scientific health article you pick up today will say something to the effect of, 'Chronic inflammation is the cause of chronic disease.' So it makes sense that if we wanted to tackle chronic disease, we must first handle chronic inflammation, right?" Joey stopped and looked for our agreement. "That," he said, "is our objective!

"And if we are going to handle chronic inflammation, we need to understand what causes it. Well, the cat's out of the bag on this, as I will be going over this whole subject thoroughly in the following weeks. You will also understand that toxins in and around our body are the culprits. "*Toxins, toxicity*!" He repeated as he wrote the word at the bottom of the board. "If we can remove toxins from the body through safe and effective detoxification methods and provide the nutrients necessary to help our stem cells rebuild our body, we can handle chronic inflammation. And if we can handle chronic inflammation, we can open the door to handling chronic disease!

It all has become very apparent that all chronic diseases and often their treatments lead to Peripheral Neuropathy.

"For the next several weeks, we will be discussing exactly what these toxins are, where they come from, why our bodies can no longer eliminate them, what they have been doing to our health, and how, by removing them, we can regain our vitality, health, and longevity."

Judy and I wiggled in our chairs as we exchanged glances. This guy was good. He was so passionate in his delivery that I figured he could singlehandedly save the world. And I was in – I had not felt this excited about anything for years, if ever. This made total sense, and I was on the edge of my seat, waiting for more.

"Not more than five years ago," Joey began, "my father sat in the exact space you are sitting in today. He, too, was wheelchair-bound but recovering from his second limb amputation. I watched for ten years as his health failed. Diabetes and the effects of its slow progression of peripheral neuropathy are what took him, and there was nothing Western Medicine had to offer him but drugs, more drugs, and then finally, surgeries to keep the gangrene away. It finally got him, though – blood poisoning took him in the middle of the night.

"They said it was a fluke, that they usually catch it soon enough. The bed sores did their share in disguising it.

"I'm sorry to get so graphic, but I think that if you don't take this seriously and dramatically change your life, your time will be short and miserable on this planet. All I can do is give you all I have, and it's up to you to make the change. I'm determined to help my mom, even if I have to fight Alice the whole time."

I looked at Joey and then at Judy and felt a wave of emotions I had not felt in years. I felt that I was part of something. I had been alone for so long, sitting in quiet desperation, allowing the health of my body to slowly decline. Again, I felt a wave of hope surge through me as I looked at my new friends and realized that, for the first time in many years, I had hope.

With all the gratitude I could muster, I looked at Joey and said, "Thank you, Joey."

With that, Joey continued. "What I am going to tell you is so current in the health science field that it will be years before traditional medicine catches on – even longer if the pharmaceutical industry has anything to say about it.

"I was fortunate enough to accompany my chiropractor to a seminar put on by a group of doctors called Health Centers of the Future. At that seminar, I was introduced to several healthcare practitioners who were studying and implementing the techniques I am teaching you today: Dr. Dan Pompa, who you will hear quite a bit about; a biochemist named Dr. Sean Morris; and a nephrologist named Dr. Jason Fung and others. These guys blew my mind. They talked about 'turning back your biological clock' and how you could reverse the aging process by removing the cause of chronic inflammation from the body. They drove home the concept that chronic inflammation was at the core of chronic disease and that the cause of chronic inflammation was exposure and absorption of toxins, whether environmental or created as biological end-products of your body's metabolism. Metabolism, meaning the processes the body goes through when burning fuel to sustain life."

I guess Joey could see my eyes begin to roll back in my head as my mind started to wander.

"Hang in there, guys," he remarked. "This sounds crazy, but I promise it will make sense to you in just a few minutes."

He handed out a sheet of paper titled "Glossary of Terms." As he erased the whiteboard, he stated,

"I'll be going over a lot of new concepts, so this glossary will be helpful for you to refer to as we work our way through the class."

*(Find the Glossary of terms in the end of the book.)*

"We need to understand why so many Americans are sick. Eighty million Americans are said to have multiple chronic diseases, according to an article coming from Michigan State University. How many Americans may have just one chronic disease? According to the CDC, 40% of our children are now diagnosed with some chronic disease. Almost any magazine article or study you pick up talks about chronic disease and how chronic inflammation is at the heart of it. Chronic inflammation is the villain, yet the lion's share of the medical model's focus is on covering up symptoms, to the tune of 4.3 trillion dollars annually. Wouldn't it make sense to find out what is causing all this chronic inflammation? If we could find the source of chronic inflammation and remove it, would that help reverse the epidemic of chronic disease we see in this country?"

With that, Joey brought our attention back to the whiteboard and said, "So, let me rewrite these words to make more sense."

"I want to get right to the point and explain how chronic inflammation occurs and how it affects your health."

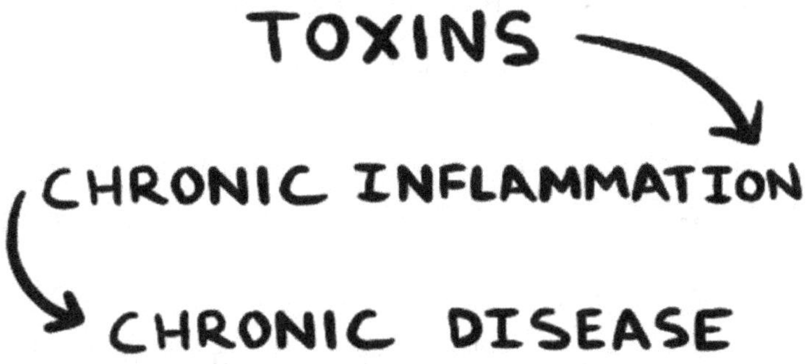

*Picture 5*

# Some Basic Tenets of Health

He looked at us and said, "Now, you are going to understand what true health is all about and what needs to happen to restore your own health. There are a few premises that we need to discuss, understand, and embrace in order for you to take charge of your health."

He asked us to follow along on the handouts he gave, and then he began to read down the list.

1. *"The power that made the body can heal the body.* This basic chiropractic philosophy – that the body has a built-in innate intelligence – goes back to D.D. Palmer, who discovered chiropractic back in 1895. However, we hear these words echoed down through the ages all the way back to Socrates and Hippocrates. These thoughts were voiced by such greats as Thomas Edison and even Benjamin Franklin.

2. *The body needs no help; it just needs no interference.* The late great Reggie Gold was a chiropractor who taught others in his profession the concept

of "The body needs no help; it just needs no inter-ference." He suggested that by removing interfer-ence from the body – be it nerve interference, chemical imbalances or toxicity, or even mental, emotional, or spiritual imbalances – we allow for healing to take place.

3. *Fix the cell to get well.* This is a phrase coined by Dr. Dan Pompa. With advances in science, the healthcare industry has discovered that this prem-ise reigns supreme. By the time we are done, you will have a good understanding of the human cell, how mapping the human DNA and its genes changed healthcare forever, and how environmen-tal factors both in and around our bodies influence our overall health and well-being.

"Okay, everybody, I think that is enough information for one day. Tonight, I want to prepare a nice, organic, keto-friendly dinner. Let's take a break to freshen up and meet back in the kitchen in an hour, and I will demonstrate how to make killer chicken curry. Does that sound good to everyone?" (The recipe is on the back of the book.)

We all agreed happily. It was quite a first day – lots of information. This would require a major shift in my thinking, but Joey seemed to understand that and was taking us through it step by step and didn't seem to mind us slogging along as we were coming up to speed.

We all assembled in the kitchen about an hour later and helped Joey chop up the ingredients for the chicken curry dish. I must say, it was fantastic. He had all these great condiments to add on top of each bite – things like organic shredded coconut, chopped cashews and almonds, diced jalapenos, green onions, and even a few cranberries. It was delicious.

We mostly ate in silence, no doubt contemplating the day's teachings but also filling the void in our stomach created partly from the anticipation of the fasting yet to come.

That evening, I lay in bed wondering how to pull this off. Still, I also felt grateful for the Jones family and the kindness and friendship they allowed me.

The next morning, we all worked our way into the kitchen for what we learned was a keto-friendly breakfast. It consisted of poached eggs on half an avocado garnished with fresh basil, and there was organic, sulfite-free bacon to boot.

I was also handed a cup of what Joey called "keto coffee." He explained that it was brewed from organic, shade-grown coffee beans and topped off with organic whipping cream. Hum… It actually tasted great, but I felt guilty drinking whipping cream. Wasn't that fattening?

We all visited and discussed what we had covered the day before. Joey said that we should take the rest of the day, absorb what we learned, and meet up next week. That sounded good to me. I actually wanted to spend some time with Judy anyway.

At her suggestion, the two of us took a drive down the Big Sur coast. It was a beautiful day. We stopped along the way, parking the car off the road and enjoying a picnic lunch Joey prepared.

It was nice to just talk and get to know her. She asked about my family. I felt comfortable enough to tell her I hadn't seen them in years and hoped to see them again someday. She reached out and touched my hand, saying that she would love to see that happen and was sure it would one day.

# CHAPTER 4

# Who's Sitting on the Three-Legged Stool

Judy again graciously invited me to come on Friday night, so I was well-rested for Saturday's class. When I arrived at Judy's house, Alice and Joey were already there, sitting with their mom in the garden. It was a pleasant midsummer afternoon, and the warm air spoke of the Pacific Ocean, which I could hear making itself known on the white sands of Carmel Beach.

That evening, Judy arranged for us to eat on the Monterey Wharf. Joey approved of the venue but did advise us on what choices we had off the menu. Nevertheless, it was a pleasant evening listening to the kids, grown though they were, banter back and forth about growing up together. I must say, though, that it did make me a bit homesick for my family, wherever they may be.

I had a great night's sleep. As I found my way to the kitchen area that next morning, anticipating a nice breakfast, I was met by Joey, who had what I recognized to be a glucose meter in his hand. He told me to stick out my finger so he could prick to it to get a blood sample and that he would check my blood glucose and ketones (*Whatever ketones are,* I thought).

Then he handed me my 'keto coffee' and said that this was breakfast and that we would have our first meal at about 12:00 p.m. Now, we ate dinner at 6:00 p.m. the night before. I'd not skipped a meal purposely since I was a kid.

When I suggested to Joey I was going to starve to death, he paused, looking at my giant belly, and said, "I think you will live, my friend!" I heard Judy stifle a chuckle as she descended the stairs from her bedroom.

As we settled in for our lesson of the day, savoring our "breakfast," Joey scribbled something on the whiteboard.

Joey began to explain that today, we were starting on a seven-week fasting journey. He called this the Cellular Healing Lifestyle Diet. He said it was a course in itself and that we would be incorporating it into our class along with other principles he would introduce us to.

He mentioned that the whipping cream is all fat and that we are going to teach our body how to use fat as fuel. By teaching it to burn ketones, our body would start burning its stored fat for fuel. He said that ketones burn very clean, like a gas stove, and that glucose burns very dirty, like a fireplace filled with wet pine wood. Because glucose burned so dirty, it was causing our body to become inflamed and contributing to the terrible health of the population. "So, hang in there," he said.

As he passed out the worksheet for today, he asked how we all did that week. He wanted us to report on how many times we put food in our mouths and how we did eating off of the keto shopping list.

We all gave our wins on how it went. It seemed I was not the only one who struggled a bit with no bread. I expressed this fact and mentioned that if it wasn't for Judy and I had talked on the phone quite a bit and helped each other through the hard times, I probably would have succumbed to my bread-eating desires.

I could see Alice and Joey glance at each other with a fun and knowing look on their faces. I was a bit embarrassed yet happy at the same time.

Joey began. "As I mentioned in our last class, each week we meet, I will start by introducing another step in the Cellular Healing Lifestyle course. This will help your body convert to burning ketones easily, which will help your body burn your fat stores and start detoxing your body.

"This week," Joey continued, "the magic begins. Your body will begin to become fat-adapted! The main thing here is that we are going to train your body to eat less often. When you eat less often, your body becomes comfortable with less food.

"Studies show people who eat less live longer! People learn to eat less by eating less often. Eating less often allows your body to become more keto-adapted, burning your stored fat. At the same time, conserve energy. A tremendous amount of your energy is used to digest your meals. Thinks about that big Holiday dinner you ate and how all you could do was lay on the couch until it was digested. So, by changing your eating patterns, what, when, and how much you eat, you allow your body to spend that unspent energy on more important things, such as healing your gut, detoxifying your liver, or healing your brain.

"Just imagine if you made a habit of eating less often, which meant you also eat less, how much more energy your body would have to heal things in your body! Plus, you'd have less brain fog, clearer focus, and get more done!" Wow, what a cool concept.

"Have you ever heard this before?" Joey asked rhetorically. "Neither had I," he said, answering his own question.

"Sign me up," I volunteered excitedly. "I need all of those things."

There was a bit of laughter, but I could tell everyone was thinking the same as me.

"You are worth it," Joey said, "and with guided support during the Cellular Healing Lifestyle program, you will find it is easy to adopt these changes! Sometimes, you just need a guiding hand.

"Today," Joey continued, "I will cover what Dr. Dan Pompa calls the three-legged stool and how your body survives in the world you live in. I will also cover the three major causes of stress in your body. I like to refer to them as the three major stressors, just so you know. These stressors act in and around your body, affecting what's called your microbiome, intestinal flora, and other bacteria that surround and cover your entire body. We have something like 75 trillion human cells in our body. These all work in coordination, sustaining life while existing in an environment that can be both nurturing and hostile. Yet homo sapiens have survived the test of time. Soon, you will understand what microbiomes are and that 100 trillion of them live in our gut alone (yes, there are more bugs in our gut than human cells in our body). These microbiomes digest our food for us and convert the food into digestible nutrients that can be absorbed into our body to sustain and forward life. We will explore how these microorganisms, both friendly and hostile, living in and around us, can either enhance or threaten our survival by promoting the expression of both 'good' and 'bad' genes. I will explain to you how the expression of these genes results in the turning on or turning off of many disease processes. These three stressors can affect the direction of all actions in your organs and cells. They can directly affect your gene expression, resulting in the turning on of bad genes which can, thus, result in disease."

With that, Joey drew the stool out on the whiteboard.

"This is Dr. Pompa's three-legged stool. By understanding this stool, you will begin to understand how and why the health of this country – your health included – has gone on the decline. As we look to each leg, we will learn how to improve the quality of each, culminating in a much better understanding of how to be and stay healthy."

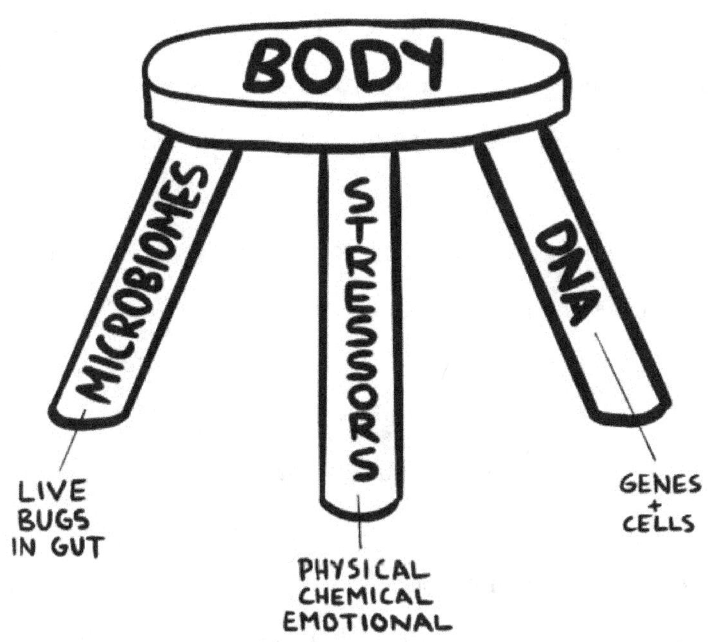



*Picture 6: The three-legged stool*

"So, I'm sure we could debate who we are, what we are, and what this thing called life is. But for today, let's agree that there is an innate intelligence that seems to animate us. We can say that some life essence seems to hang around the body as long as it is inhabitable. Of course, once the body ceases to be livable, for whatever reason, this innate intelligence seems to leave the body and go… who knows where.

"This life essence seems to think a thought. Then, by enlisting emotion, it puts the game of life into actual motion. The most primitive example of turning emotion into motion is the 'fight or flight' mechanism, which we will discuss in detail shortly. But for now, I'll give the example of being startled. This creates an endocrine/ hormone response as adrenaline pours into your bloodstream from your adrenal glands, allowing for superhuman strength. We've all seen or heard about this as mom picks up the car with one hand to save her baby.

On a higher level of survival, someone can have a dream to be or do something; the emotions involved with even the hope or the actual attainment of that dream can be very powerful. Only you have the power of choice, of goal setting, of attaining that goal, of unwavering determination, and of the ability to reach for the stars or decay into dust. Whatever drives you to greatness or mediocrity seems to exist in the realm of create, exist, and decay. Many decisions you made along the way put you exactly where you are and in the condition you are in today. There are many outside influences: toxins, anaerobes, climates, neighbors, and governments, including their agencies, which also affect your state of health and push you toward prosperity, poverty, freedom, or slavery.

"Logic tells us that if we want to enjoy our time on this planet, we should keep this vehicle called the body running as smoothly and efficiently as possible for as long as possible, keeping all its parts well maintained. Even though this may seem logical as it also seems logical to keep your car well maintained or your home clean and safe, many people don't seem to heed the call, and so let any or all of these possessions, from homes, vehicle, and even their body, to go to Hell in a hand basket.

"Many people won't be able to see these things clearly enough to make a decision to thrive but, rather, continue stuck somewhere between boredom, playing the victim, or sheer apathy. For me, I'd rather die trying to shoot for the stars than roll over in defeat. How about you? What is it about one person versus another that allows each individual to survive, and to survive at what level? What drives each one of us toward our dreams and goals or, maybe too often, holds us back from even dreaming dreams in the first place?"

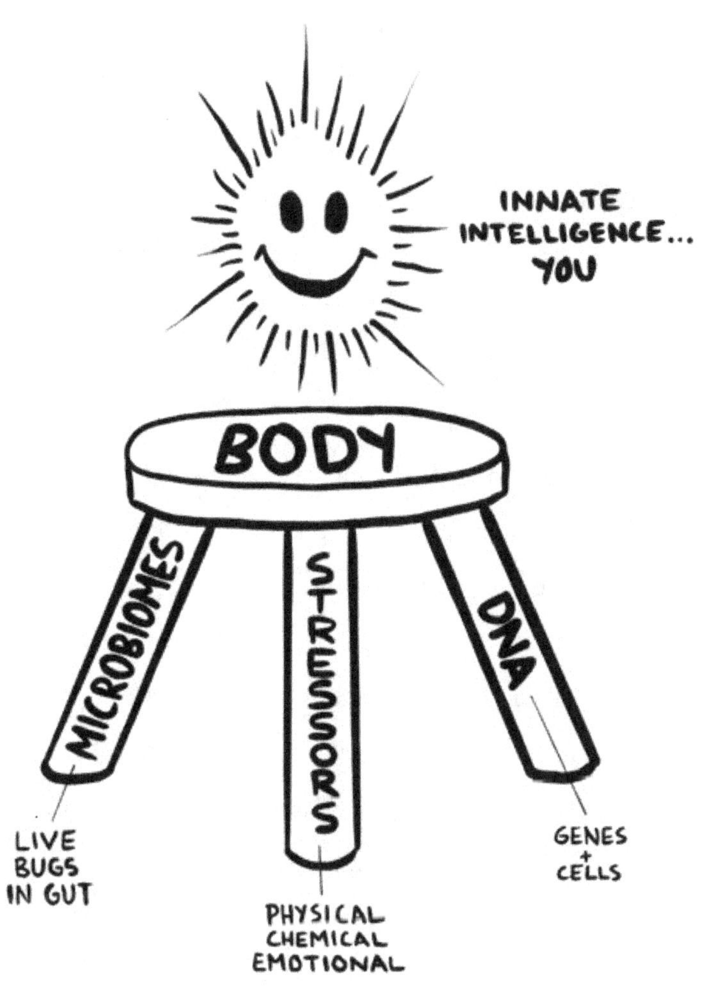


*Picture 7: Innate intelligence and the three-legged stool*

119

Joey then added a smiley face on top of the three-legged stool, indicating it to represent innate intelligence or life itself.

"At the end of the day, the choice is only yours to make. If you don't decide to change, no drug, vitamin, surgery, potion, or snake oil in the world will help!"

"I am pushing this concept here because I want to see you succeed or die in the attempt."

Joey walked over to the table, unscrewed the top of his water bottle, and proceeded to guzzle all its contents.

"Sorry, I didn't mean to climb up on my soapbox. But there you go: emotion being converted into action!

"Okay, so now that we know who's sitting on it, let's break down the three-legged stool. At the top of the stool is considered the body, and each leg represents one of three major aspects of your health. Each leg interplays with the others. If one side goes down or becomes unhealthy or damaged, it will have an adverse effect on the other two legs. Conversely, by strengthening any of the legs, we can improve the overall health of the body.

"Let's take a look at each of these three legs and see what they are and how we can optimize each.

"The left leg represents the microbiome or bugs (bacteria, viruses, microbes, parasites, molds, etc.) that exist in and around us. As I said, they either work with us to help us survive or work against us to make us sick."

"The middle leg represents the three major stressors: physical, chemical, and mental. We will go over them in detail a bit later."

"The right leg represents our human DNA."

## The Right Leg DNA (your genes and their expression)

I'm sure you recall from High School science class that Deoxyribonucleic Acid exists in the nucleus of every cell in your body, making up 23 pairs of chromosomes, 46 individual chromosomes, 23 from each parent make up a pair. These chromosomes comprise the 20,000-25,000 genes that make up the human body, holding your genetic coding and unique operating instructions. Genes are passed down from your parents; they express your characteristics. They also may dictate the expression of genetic disease should they be 'turned on,' thus threatening your survival. Keywords 'turned on,' which implies that they can also be 'turned off' as well. Toxins in the cell can turn on these bad genes expressing disease. By detoxing the body and lowering the toxic level inside the cell and its nucleus, we can effect "turning off' the bad genes. Shortly, we will watch a short video by Dr. Bruce Lipton illustrating this concept.

So, the toxic buildup in the cell can turn on bad genes, and removing the toxins from the cells can turn off the bad genes is the premise. This is as easy as it gets," Joey continued. "If you get this concept and apply it, you will have a pretty good understanding of what you need to know to overcome the chronic or age-related diseases plaguing you and, quite honestly, our nation if not the world."

"But for now," Joey paused, "I think we need to feed our brains. It's time for lunch!"

Hurrays and yays erupted from the group. And I realized that I was starving.

Lucky for us, Joey anticipated our empty stomach and prepared broiled chicken breasts dusted with salt and pepper and a touch of cumin and chili powder. They were delicious. They were served with an arugula salad topped with roasted pecans and sliced Granny Smith apples. He also allowed for a smallish portion of baked sweet potato. I loved that he said we could use all the butter we wanted and recommended being liberal with the olive or avocado oil on our salad.

After lunch, we visited for a few minutes before returning to work. It felt so lovely to be part of a family again. After my wife died, I just seemed to drift into being a hermit. Wow, it's hard to see how people just let life happen and end up sick and unhappy.


## The Left Leg, the Microbiome

After a nice break to get some fresh air, Joey beckoned us back to class.

"So now, the left leg of the stool represents not only all the 100,000 microbiome or live bugs that live within our digestive system – specifically our intestines – but also the exponential number of microbiomes that live on this planet. We are surrounded by them. We can't live without them. What is so amazing and only recently understood is that the health of our intestinal friends directly affects our body's health. If our intestinal microbiome or bacteria are unbalanced or sick, we are, too. If they are healthy, we have a chance.

"The microbiome can generally be divided into three classes: those that digest carbohydrates, those that digest protein, and those that digest fats.

"In the digestive track of today's average American, there is a plethora of each – some healthy, some not so healthy. Think of an unkept garden; it might have some pretty flowers, but will eventually be overrun with weeds. In the case of your digestive tract, these would be the unhealthy microbiome. As I mentioned the other day, various lifestyles, diets, habits, medications, illnesses, etc. stress the good bacteria. The careless use of antibiotics over the years not only weakened our immune system by wiping out the majority of healthy microbiomes but also created resistant strains of bad bacteria. These bacteria are smart, and just like us, they have the goal to survive, so they mutate and adapt. Today, because of these microbiome's ability to adapt, many antibiotics don't even work anymore. There are resistant strains of bacteria that can't be touched, especially in hospitals.

"Currently and quite honestly, since the Second World War, we have seemingly unlimited food resources. In other words, we could basically eat what we want, when we want, wherever we want, with whomever we want, and as much as we want with little scrutiny.

"This 'freedom' based on the world climate variations allowed us to have ripe melon from South America in the dead of winter or fresh spinach in January. On the surface, this seems like a good thing, but really, it never allows for a challenge of your digestive system or stress to the microbiome in your gut. As a result, our microbiome becomes lazy and doesn't have to adapt to the season. Our defenses go down, and so does our body's ability to handle stress.

**Hormesis**

There is a term called 'hormesis,' which I think is important to introduce here. You can look it up yourself later, but basically, hormesis describes how a bit of stress that acts on your body can help build up a better resistance to that substance and the environment. This is how Homeopathy works. You give a bit of a toxin to the patient, which causes the body to overcome the toxin, creating a resistance to it. If you give too much too fast, it could kill the patient. But a little bit over time builds your immune response. Think of the kid who grew up in a protected, sterile environment versus little Jonny, who grew up on the farm playing with all the farm animals and playing outside in the dirt all day. Who do you think has a stronger immune system?

**Diet Variation**

My main point here is diet variation, which I will expound on later. Diet variation, historically, was the result of what could be grown during what season in any given geographic location. This created a seasonal diversity of foods, which had a hermetic effect (hormesis) on our intestinal microbiome, keeping the good, strong microbiome alive while starving off the weaker and unhealthy ones.

We will explore diet variation more as we move along, but I wanted to touch on it today. Diet variation using the correct healthy foods creates a hermetic effect on our body. One thing you will learn to implement in the future is the continued practice of diet variation.

"Since approximately 70% of our immune system is found in our digestive tract, an unhealthy GI tract can dramatically lower the immune response and be devastating health-wise.

"So, by practicing the cellular healing lifestyle, including all the five steps we teach –

- *intermittent fasting*
- *ketogenic diet*
- *diet variation*
- *ancient healing strategies*
- *and cellular detoxification*

you can expect to see your health improve rapidly and systematically."

"These five aspects of your Cellular Healing Lifestyle program will help to reset your intestinal microbiome, establishing a healthy environment and a healthier proportion of the different types of microbiomes in your digestive tract. This will help your body's immune system knock out the interlopers, the invaders, the opportunistic anaerobes

(non-oxygen-using bugs in your body), or any other weakened gut occupants, which only further disease and ill
health.”

“As this happens, your intestinal wall will heal, and the
chronic inflammation throughout your body will begin to
subside. Then, your body can start to heal itself.”

“Now, remember when I mentioned autophagy? By intermittent fasting, which I will explain in detail as we go,
your body will begin to starve out the unhealthy microbiome. There is less food to go around, so only the strong
survive. The good news is that the strong, healthy microbiomes and your strengthening immune system will target
the bad microbiome and begin to wipe them out. By not
consuming ‘enough’ foodstuff while doing a fast, your
body will actually target these bad guys and eat them for
fuel. Pretty cool, yes?”

“Now, as we shift from one food type to the other
(carbs, protein, or fat), your body breaks down the type of
food not getting fed. For example, suppose we are on a
high-fat diet – as in keto – the carb-loving, as well as the
protein-loving. In that case, microbiomes don’t get enough

to eat, and the weak ones fade while the strong ones survive. As we apply *diet variation* and shift to a high-protein diet – as in, say, paleo, which we won't go into at this point because I'm mentioning it as an example – and if we shift the foods to high-protein, low-fat, and lower carbs, the same thing happens. The weaker ones fade into the food-deprived group, and the strong survive."

"So, you begin to see how vital diet variation can be in changing and improving your health. I want you to understand that as we reestablish a healthy microbiome in our gut, they will digest our food and make healthy byproducts that pass through the wall of our intestinal track into our bloodstream and our cells to create life."

"By the way, the unhealthy bacteria that have accumulated in our digestive tract and throughout our body over time eat our foodstuff and poop toxins known as mycotoxins. These things are deadly over time because they cause chronic inflammation and chronic disease."

**Hidden Infections**

"These bad microbiomes can take up residence in the many dark areas of our body; staying hidden; and slowly secrete their poop, excrement, or mycotoxins insidiously into our body. Here, we have the source of *hidden infections,* which can be difficult to detect or locate. Mainstream medicine does not look for these, and some philosophies argue their existence. A large portion of these bad guys can be hidden in the root canals, jaw bones, or gums. If they go undetected, it can be close to impossible to heal from some of the plethora of *autoimmune* diseases America suffers from, many of which are often brushed off as 'all in your head' by some doctors. But worry not. There is hope in the hands of people who know their signs and symptoms and how to locate and remove them. You can be helped. These bad guys can be located anywhere in the body. They may exist as a fungus in your toes, a cavitation in a root canal, or an infection in your elbow."

## Middle Leg Stressors (Physical, Chemical, Emotional/Mental)

"These three stressors create both good and harmful effects on your body. When they become acutely overwhelming or constant and chronic, they can produce the 'fight or flight' mechanism, which automatically shuts down or lowers your digestive function. So, the middle leg of this three-legged stool messes up your digestion and allows bad microbiomes or bacteria (and other bad guys) to grow in your intestine. This allows bad things to get into your body and into your cells.

1. **Physical** - You can have nerve interruption (subluxation or pinched nerve) to the organs or systems involved in the detox pathways, such as the lymphatic, circulatory, or digestive (liver – major detox organ) system.

2. **Chemical** - You can have chemical stressors created by your body's own systems or from exposure to the tremendous amount of toxins in your environment.

3. **Mental/Emotional** - You can have mental/ emotional stressors created either by your own mind, others, or by the challenges of life itself.

"Any and all of these three stressors can shut down your digestive, immune, cognitive as well as other systems in your body."

"I will cover these thoroughly in another lesson, so for now, just understand what they are."

"So, now you can see that you have several things affecting your body and your well-being. You will learn about the stored toxins (heavy metals, molds, biochemical) you accumulated over your lifetime, as well as the toxic load your mother unknowingly passed on to you during her pregnancy. All of these toxins are predominantly stored in your fat cells. On top of that, you most likely have sluggish organs, kind of like a dirty vacuum filter, clogged oil or air filter, or even a full lint catcher on your dryer. All these play a role in your detox pathways and overall health."

"All of the above stressors add fuel to the inflammatory fire, impacting our survival."

"I want you to know that something can be done about it. There are many different approaches to getting your health back. We will be implementing many of them as we go along. We will implement others later as they apply to you individually."

"Today, there are so many remarkable technologies, therapies, and treatments, from corrective chiropractic care to stem cell machines, stem cell injection, cellular healing diets, ketogenic diets, paleo diets, different types of fasting cellular detoxification, and more. So, with dedication, a desire to change, and a bit of hard work, you have a tremendous opportunity to get your health and, thus, your life back!"

"The next subject I want to go over with you will be how stress from any of the three stressors affects cell function and how cells become inflamed and cease to function correctly. This is a big subject, so I want to ensure we are fresh when we review it. Just so you are prepared, we will be discussing the cell wall and cell function in detail and what needs to be done to ensure that the existence of any of these is not causing you to stay ill. We will come up with solutions once these are uncovered, so hang in there. We have a lot to do!"

"But for today, that's all I have. Let's go enjoy ourselves and see what dinner brings."

"By the way, I just want to congratulate you on your first day of intermittent fasting. Since we ate last night at 6:00 p.m. and did not have lunch until 12:00 p.m. today, you completed a twelve-hour intermittent fast! And what is cool is that you didn't even realize it!"

Joey was right. Somehow, I didn't get very hungry before lunch, and then lunch seemed to fill me up and hold me over pretty well. When I mentioned that, Judy and Alice also spoke up, confirming similar experiences to mine.

"This is great," Joey said. "You all spent the last seven days eating only three meals a day and as close to keto-friendly as you could. This tells me that all of you are already converting over to burning ketones. It will be fun to check in the morning and see what your readings are. I'm proud of all of you!"

When we all assembled in the kitchen after taking some time to enjoy the garden, rest, or do whatever seemed right, Joey was already pulling dinner out of the fridge. On tonight's menu was braised skirt steak, steamed asparagus (slathered in butter), portabella mushrooms sautéed in coconut oil and ghee seasoned with a dash of cumin and ground, roasted fennel seeds, with a butter lettuce salad sprinkled with goat cheese, avocado oil, and red wine vinegar.

It was amazing, filling, and immensely satisfying. That evening, we all watched an old movie and hit the hay early.

That was quite a bit of information to be taken in by our nonscientific minds.

# CHAPTER 5

# Fix The Cell To Get Well

When I woke up Sunday morning, I realized I was feeling better than I had for years. I completely transitioned out of the wheelchair mid-last week and was beginning to master the crutches. I decided to see if I could get by on one today. Moving around a bit in my bedroom gave me the confidence I needed. It felt good to move around a bit, and I didn't feel quite so helpless.

As I worked my way into the kitchen, I could see that I was the late arrival. Joey met me with what he called his Keto Mojo Meter to test my glucose and ketones. I was used to testing my glucose, being a diabetic and all, but I never knew anything about testing for ketones. After pricking my finger – I called it bloodletting – he took my readings. He got excited and said that my glucose was still high but in a much better range. What really got him going was that my ketone reading was at 2.0. He noted that it was a good number, that I was already in ketosis, and that my body was becoming a good fat burner. Judy's test showed her at 0.5 and Alice at 0.4. Joey said that I got the gold star for the day! This, of course, drew a laugh from the group. He said that we would learn more about ketosis as we progressed in the course.

As I sipped on my morning breakfast of organic, shade-grown, freshly ground French roasted coffee with a half-inch of organic whipping cream in it, I reflected on the events of the last three weeks. I marveled at how luck had landed me in a hospital room with Judy. I felt so fortunate and wondered what my life would have been like if I hadn't met her and her family. I'd probably be back in my apartment alone, watching some stupid TV show, eating pizza, and drinking beer against doctor's orders.

We were beginning to settle in when Alice approached me. "Fred," she somewhat whispered, "I just want to thank you for being here. Your friendship with my mom really affected her outlook on life. Since you two met in the hospital room, my mom changed. I see a spark in her that has not been there for years, even since before my father died. I love my mother, Fred, and if there is anything I can do to make her happy for the rest of her life, I'd do it, even if it means following my little brother's stupid diet!" She winked. "Thank you for being here!"

Judy was just approaching the chair next to mine. As she began to sit, I could feel that she scooted her chair over a bit so that our hands were almost touching. I could feel the excitement of new love in the air. Finally, Judy placed her hand on top of mine, and then, looking into my eyes, she mouthed, "Thank you."

I could feel a glow of excitement as she did so. Life seemed to say, "I'm yours for the taking. Come and get me," yet there was also a tiny whisper of a voice that said, "Forget it, Fred. Just give up. What are you thinking any-way?" Yet I could not remember feeling so excited about my life for many years. I felt like a kid in class waiting for the school bell to ring so I could go ask Judy for a date. I could not believe my good fortune. As I could feel the warmth coming off of Judy's hand so close to mine, I could not help but reach over and gently clasp it. I could feel a contraction in her hand as she gently ensured me by her touch that she welcomed mine.

Joey stepped up to the board, clearing his throat as if ringing the school bell and announcing that class was about to begin.

"Okay," Joey stated, "are we ready to get going?"

We all agreed we were; he wasted no time jumping back into it.

"So, as a review of yesterday, based on the three-legged model we covered," Joey proclaimed, "the middle leg consists of the stressors. There are three of them – physical, chemical, and emotional/ spiritual – and they have a huge effect on the microbiome inside your body, the left leg, specifically your gut, but around your body as well. These three stressors have a huge impact on your body's cells that, of course, house your DNA and genes on the right leg.

"Thus, as a consequence and adverse effect of this overload of stressors, 'bad' genes are activated, expressing themselves in your body as acute or chronic, genetics-related diseases.

"By following this logic, then, through the 'reverse engineering' of this process, we should be able to heal the cell walls by removing or reducing the toxic build-up they accumulated from the three stressors and, while consuming healthy foods and nutrients and avoiding new toxins as much as possible, our innate intelligence can repair the damage to the cell walls, thus allowing for the propagation of new healthier cells. Then, based on earlier expressed statements from some leaders in healthcare, going as far back as Hippocrates and Socrates – let alone B.J. Palmer, Dr. Dan Pompa, and Dr Reggie Gold – the body should do what it does best: heal itself!

"Remember, your body has an innate intelligence designed to be and stay healthy and to, above all, survive. And so, having survived for millennia, this innate intelligence might yet have the ability to help us heal and survive again – that is, as long as we can remove enough toxins from it and from its environment while at the same time feeding it the right nutrients and fuel."

With that, Joey drew a big circle on the whiteboard.

"This is where Dr. Dan Pompa comes in."

"Let's say this is a human cell. We have something like seventy-five trillion of them. They are the only living part of our body. Think of the line of the circle as the cell border or cell wall. This cellular membrane allows or prohibits things like hormones, vitamins, minerals, enzymes, toxins, and other substances from entering, exiting, or acting on the cell. According to Dr. Bruce Lipton, these cell membranes are the most intelligent part of the human body."

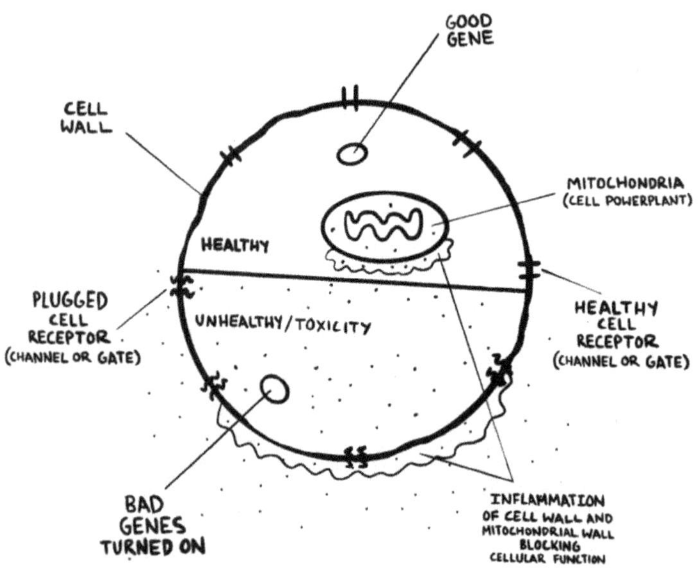


*Picture 8: The cell*

As your cells still attempt to convert fuel (glucose and ketones) into energy, they continue to create their own exhaust during cellular energy production, called cellular debris. All these things – combined with all the external toxins that accumulate in your body – culminate in plugged cell receptors on the cell walls, making it difficult for the body to utilize hormones, neurotransmitters, vitamins, and minerals or burn clean energy. As the body struggles to keep up with the demands of living, organs, and systems start to fail – usually the least life-threatening first. These usually appear as mild to moderate symptoms, typically 'handled' with a drug, herb, medication, or supplement in an attempt to make the symptoms go away. When the body's detoxification functions or systems become overly stressed and are unable to sufficiently clean these toxins out of your cells and body, more chronic inflammation occurs. Eventually, if not corrected, this causes more serious chronic disease. These are not limited to genetic diseases as a result of 'bad' genes.

"Eventually, the body can't handle it anymore, and one or more disease processes begin the demise of the organism."

"What happened at a toxic cellular level is that the toxins inside the cell that could not get out acted on the genes that comprise our DNA and turned the 'bad' genes on. Genes causing diseases such as Alzheimer's, multiple sclerosis, Parkinson's, rheumatoid, or any of the arthritides – you name it, you've got them. Remember, we are made up of 20,000 to 25,000 genes, so let's learn how to keep the healthy."

"So, do you remember earlier when I said that the majority of scientific data today points to chronic inflammation as the source of chronic disease? Well, there you go. And at the source of chronic inflammation is toxicity – either an accumulation of external or internal toxins."

"If you go to the medical doctor, you will probably end up with a nice diagnosis and a prescription to cover up the symptoms or manage the disease, but rarely a solution."

"Something *can* be done about it. Now, several questions may arise:

1. Where do these toxins come from?
2. How do we prevent or minimize further exposure to them?
3. How do we repair the damage done?

4. How do we prevent this from happening in the future?

5. How can we reestablish proper cellular energy and organ function?

"We will spend the next several days working on various aspects of handling these questions."

"In the meantime, let's take a break. When we come back, we will break down the three stressors and the middle leg of the stool!"

"But first," Joey said, "it's time to open up our eating window. Let's eat."

You never had to say that phrase twice around this group. We were up and at 'em almost before he finished his sentence.

Lunch was a beautiful salad from a local organic restaurant. It consisted of roasted chicken breasts cooked in olive oil and rosemary and veggies – carrots, yellow squash of some kind, and yellow onions – sautéed in butter and coconut oil and seasoned with sage and thyme. For dessert, we had a small bowl of coconut yogurt with a few organic local blackberries on top.

# CHAPTER 6

# The Three Stressors

We eagerly gathered back to the den after lunch. I was noticing that rather than being hit with the after-meal drowsiness I thought was normal, I actually felt energized. I mentioned as much to Joey, and Judy and Alice immediately concurred.

"That is what happens when you feed your body brain food rather than the standard American diet most people eat on a regular basis. That diet is typically filled with toxic grains, including all the pesticides, herbicides, additives, and fillers our food industry shoves down our throats. We have been programmed by TV and all forms of media that this stuff is healthy. Well, look at the results! This inflammatory diet contributed so much to the disease state of our country that it almost seems criminal. I am so happy you are all feeling so much better. And we are only three weeks into it!"

"You know what else is pretty cool, Joey?" I asked, getting everyone's attention.

"What's that?" he asked.

"I got on the scale this morning and actually lost fifteen pounds since we started," I said.

There was a cacophony of hurrays that I had to interrupt by saying, "And that's not all … I have not had to take a pain pill for two days!"

This was met with even more enthusiasm.

I had been taking Norco since the surgery. Usually, I topped it off with 800 mg of Ibuprofen twice a day, and sometimes that did not even touch the pain. So, to be off of it completely… wow!

"This is perfect timing, Fred," Joey said, "because this afternoon we are going to break down the three stressors that are affecting you and causing the chronic inflammation that has been clogging and poisoning your cells and organs and causing you to be in a chronically diseased state."

I was on the edge of my seat and could feel the energy in the room. This was not just good information – it was life-changing information. I knew it, and I knew Judy and Alice were feeling it, too.

"Okay," Joey said, "and in the words of the late Jackie Gleason, 'And away we go!' Now that you better understand how the body manages to survive on this planet, let's look at what we can do to help it along. We are about to jump into what Dr. Dan Pompa has coined as 'fix the cell to get well.' With that, I will introduce you to what Dr. Bruce Lipton describes as the most intelligent part of the human body: the cell wall. Everything we talked about so far has to do with what is happening at a cellular level.

"You heard the phrase 'the stress is killing me' before, right?" Joey asked. "Well, let me tell you, it literally is. But we need to understand that stress is a good thing, too – that is, until it overwhelms us, at which point our body and even our minds start to break down."

"Stress," Joey began, "is part of life. We need it to keep our body vibrant and to keep its defense systems strong. Stress on our muscles, like in a workout, builds up strength; stress on the immune system builds up immunity. But when one or more of the three major stressors becomes overwhelming and weakens some part of our body, we become sick, diseased, immobile, or mentally challenged. When stress becomes too overpowering, we die."

"As I mentioned earlier, stress comes in three forms: physical, chemical, and mental/emotional/spiritual. Stress shapes our lives and, even from the beginning of time, works to help us develop into the beings and bodies that we are and have, the groups that we hang out with, and even the immune system we develop."

"Physical stressors allowed for the creation of strong bones, ligaments, and muscles, as well as a durable outer layer of skin to protect us from the environment."

"Chemical stressors allowed for our amazing digestive and detoxification system so that we can consume things from the environment to burn as fuel and then eliminate the toxic byproducts."

"Mental stressors allowed for cognitive thought so that we might survive our predators, overcome the immediate problems of life, and learn to work with others to build communities, which not only protects us but also allow for a higher quality of existence."

He drew a triangle on the white board and labeled the
sides.

# THE HEALTH TRIANGLE

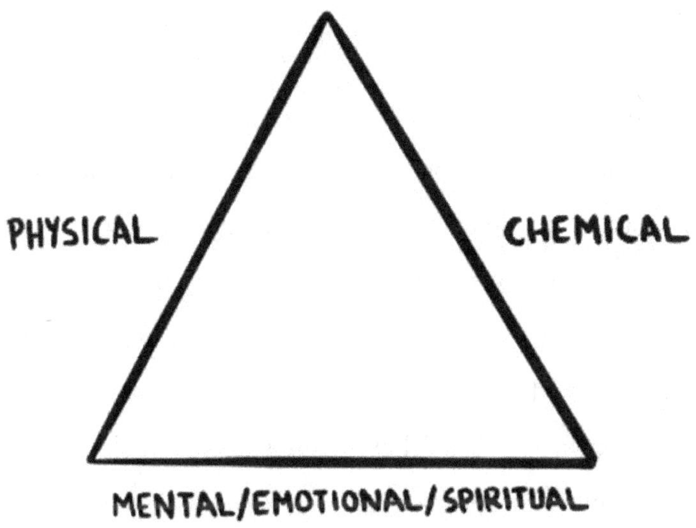


*Picture 9: The health triangle*

"The combination of these stressors can either work with you or against you. You can use your control over these stressors to enhance your body and move forward with your goals and desires. But if any or all of them become too much or overwhelming, they can have adverse effects on you and culminate in disease and visits to the infirmary." "You see," Joey continued, "if you can determine to what degree each of these three stressors is adversely affecting your current state of health and reduce or eliminate them, your body's innate intelligence – its ability to adapt to its environment and become healthy and survive – can take over and give you your life back!

"Now, I want to look at each of these three stressors and discuss what each of you can do to overcome any challenges your body has. These challenges are blocking your body's innate ability to heal."

I was becoming excited at the prospect of taking control of my life. I could feel it in Judy as well. I could also feel a deeper connection growing between us as our vitality was stirring to a higher level. I was feeling that I had a new lease on life and was looking forward to creating a future with Judy in it. I glanced at Alice, who was sitting quietly and taking in everything her brother was saying. I could tell that even she was ready for the challenge.

"These stressors accumulate in, on, and around our body and alter the functions of many systems in the body. If they accrue in too large a number, they can damage the actual organs and tissues in the body, including our brain. This particular type of stress will be a big part of what we will address to remove chronic inflammation from our body and allow the body to heal itself."

# AREAS AFFECTED BY STRESS

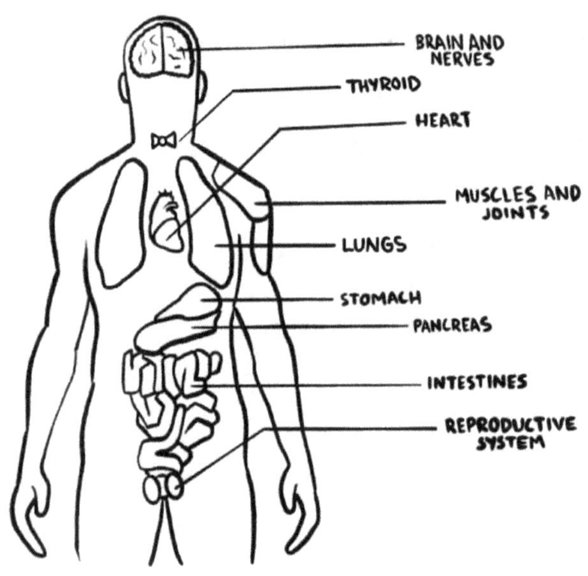



*Picture 10: Areas of the body affected by stress*

# Physical Stressors

"Even though we will spend the lion's share of the time discussing chemical and biochemical stressors and how these contributed significantly to your current state of health, I want to start with the physical stressors and how they impact us."

"Our lives outside of the womb begin with the journey down the birth canal, a process which, in itself, can be quite challenging for both the mother and child. Often times, especially in the days of forceps birth, suction, or even just difficult births alone, this voyage can cause physical trauma to the child, which can affect the child's proper development. This journey, though, is a natural phenomenon that not only inoculates the infant with the healthy bacteria in the mom's birth canal, boosting the child's immune system, but also creates stress on the skull, body, and spinal cord, which has been said to help infuse the child with adaptation reflexes. Again, hormesis and stressors challenge our survival, resulting in increased resistance to the environment. Unfortunately, today, according to the CDC, 25 to 35% of all hospital births in the U.S. are cesarean, which deprives the child of the mother's natural immunity existing in her birth canal. Instead of the birth canal bacteria, the child is first exposed to pathogens hanging around the hospital. One could argue that the children of cesarean birth have a weakened immune system to those of vaginal births."

"Of course, then we have slips, falls, accidents, and injuries from sports, work, play, or just plain living. Damage to bones, muscle, tissue, organs, and even the brain (as in concussion) – even if treated to the best of our current medical system's ability – has a lasting deleterious (injurious) effect on the body."

"Our nervous system exits our brain as the central nervous system. The CNS travels down the center of our spinal canal and exits as thirty-one pairs of spinal nerves. Once the nerves exit the spine, they are deemed the peripheral nervous system or PNS – basically because they now exist in the periphery of the spine. These thirty-one pairs of nerves split and split until they communicate with the 75 trillion human cells we are composed of. As long as this communication is intact, our body can read and adapt to the environment as information travels up and down the central nervous system and in and out of the spine via the peripheral nervous system. This is so the brain can dictate the body's safest and most pro-survival course of action to flourish and prosper. B.J. Palmer, son of D.D. Palmer, is known as the developer of chiropractic. After taking the reins from his father D.D., B.J.'s most basic tenet – the life blood of true chiropractic today – states that 'the body heals from above-down inside-out,' basically saying that the body has an innate intelligence to heal."

Joey continued, "When our bodies come in contact with the physical environment too fast – as in a whiplash, sports activity, or fall – the spinal bones can become misaligned, putting pressure on the spinal nerves and interrupting proper communication."

"Each spinal nerve travels to different organs, muscle tissue, and body systems. Pressure on just one of the sixty-two spinal nerves (thirty-one on each side) can create a myriad of effects. The presence or absence of pain is not an accurate indicator of nerve pressure or spinal misalignment. Sometimes, the pressure exerted on a nerve can only affect the organ it innervates or the associated muscle's strength and yet have no pain associated with it at all. Sometimes, it remains silent and insidiously progresses to eventually cause a symptom. This is like a cavity in your tooth – it can go undetected for years before it erupts into a wild toothache. This pain or symptom relief model has been responsible, to a large degree, for the rampant diseases our country suffers from."

"We've been taught from the get-go to eat Tums, Advil, Aspirin, Tylenol, Nexium, high-blood-pressure or cholesterol meds, metformin, asthma drugs, and more to control our symptoms without any regard to what might be at the source of the problem. This is like continuing to put air in your car's tire without looking for the nail that is causing the air to leak out. Yet when it comes to our health, this is the norm – cover up the symptoms and move on. It's no wonder we take more pharmaceutical drugs than any other country in the world. Remember, we are only 4% of the world's population, yet we take over 50% of the world's prescription consumption. So, if more drugs was the answer, we should be healthy as an ox, as the old saying goes."

"Another example – and sorry, but I really want to make sure you get this, so I want to spend a bit more time on this. If you have a cavity in your tooth which was small and asymptomatic, and you ignored it, and one day it started to get sore occasionally, and you just took aspirin and went about your day, I don't think you would be surprised if one day you woke up with a whopping tooth ache. I'm sure you would wish that you had done something sooner. Well, it is that way with our health in general. Symptoms are there to tell us something is wrong; don't ignore them."

"However, I want to clarify here so there is no misunderstanding: a lack of symptoms does not mean you are healthy either. How often do we hear a story about someone's poor old Uncle Joe who was 'as healthy as an ox,' a young man in his fifties with no symptoms at all – then one day, *bam!* He died of a heart attack. Was he 100% healthy the day before the heart attack? Or did he just have no symptoms? In our country, 50% of the time, the first sign of heart disease is death!"

"At any rate, my point here is that having as close to 100% functional communication from the brain to the body and vice versa is essential to proper health."

"People I have talked to often say, 'Oh, my doctor told me I have arthritis in my spine; that's why I'm in pain.' I want to tell you right now that the term arthritis is a waste-basket term. There are many types of arthritis – some are inflammatory, such as rheumatoid arthritis or psoriatic arthritis. Some are basically wear-and-tear from misaligned vertebra or other structural bones; this is called osteo (bony) or degenerative arthritis. So, the diagnosis of arthritis may be a diagnosis of elimination, which means nothing in some cases. Here is an example I think you can relate to. If you bought a brand-new set of tires for your car, the moment you drove out of the shop, you have tire wear. Are they bald or just slightly worn? Dr. McCollum showed me many sets of X-rays. There were examples of perfect-looking spines where the person could not walk and some spines that looked completely fused, yet the person had no symptoms. All I am saying is since this is the only body you have right now, let's make sure it is as healthy as can be. Get your spine checked, and I recommend you do so with a corrective care chiropractor – if you are interested in longevity, that is."

"You see, when bones of the spine called vertebra get knocked out of place – and this can happen from anything, a fall, mental stress, food poisoning, or sleeping wrong –

99.9% of the time, they fix themselves within two or three days without chiropractic, drugs, medicine, physical therapy, surgery, or whiskey. The problem is that maybe one in a thousand times, it does not self-correct 100%. Then, just like a tiny cavity in your tooth or a misaligned front end of your car, the condition escalates into advanced spinal degeneration (arthritis), which can be devastating not only in terms of pain but also by shutting off the proper nerve control to organs and systems in the body which that affected nerve innervates."

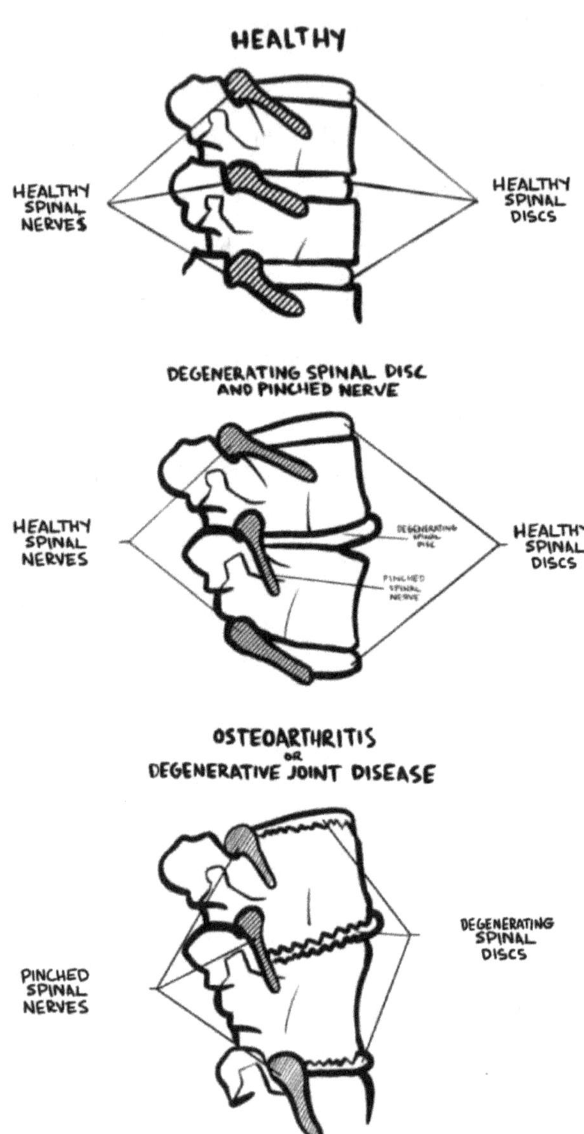


*Picture 11: Degenerating spinal disc*

"An example would be a pinched, misaligned, or *subluxated (chiropractic term for such)* bone in the neck, which can cause headaches, numbness, pain, or weakness in the neck, shoulder, arm, elbow, wrist, and hands. Also note that if this same nerve goes to the thyroid, heart, and lungs, it would make sense that pressure on this nerve could also cause disfunction of these organs, such as hyper or hypothyroid conditions, asthmas, allergies, or even heart palpitations. Another example would be what ultimately killed my dad and took your foot, Fred, peripheral neuropathy. When a nerve is damaged or interferes with exiting the spine, it will eventually start to die. The nerves in the lower spine exit and form nerves such as the sciatic nerve, which journeys down your leg and all the way to your toes. Pressure at the spinal level can affect the health of the nerve, eventually causing the nerve to cease to thrive, contributing to the nerve's demise. As a caveat, if we corrected the spinal subluxation and it caused the organic symptoms (by organic, I mean asthma, hypothyroid, etc.) to subside, it would make sense that the nerve pressure or subluxation was, in some part, responsible for the organic condition. On the other hand, if we corrected the subluxation and, in doing so, did not correct the organic condition, then it is important to look to other 'upstream' causes."

"The nerves between the shoulders innervate the stomach, gallbladder, pancreas, spleen, and other organs in the area, while the lower back is responsible for bowel function as well as that of the bladder, prostate (for men), and reproductive organs (for both sexes). Remember, though, again, you don't have to have pain in your back to think that the nerve must be affecting the organs. You could have something like colitis, Crohn's Disease, infertility or erectile disfunction, painful periods, or frequent bladder issues with absolutely no back pain. Oh, and by the way, the lower back nerves also extend down the legs to the foot and tips of your toes, so any symptoms of the lower extremities – peripheral neuropathy, sciatica, muscle weakness, numbness, or things like RLS (Restless Leg Syndrome) – should be suspect to subluxations or nerve impingement as a factor in the causative factor regarding issues in that area. *People love a diagnosis.*"

"In wrapping up the physical component of stress – at least for now – just remember that the nervous system is the number one communication system in the body. Any malfunctions in it can and usually do end up as a major factor in dysfunction and disease. Don't overlook this if you are looking to turn back your biological clock."

"Don't get caught up in the medical model of covering up your symptoms."

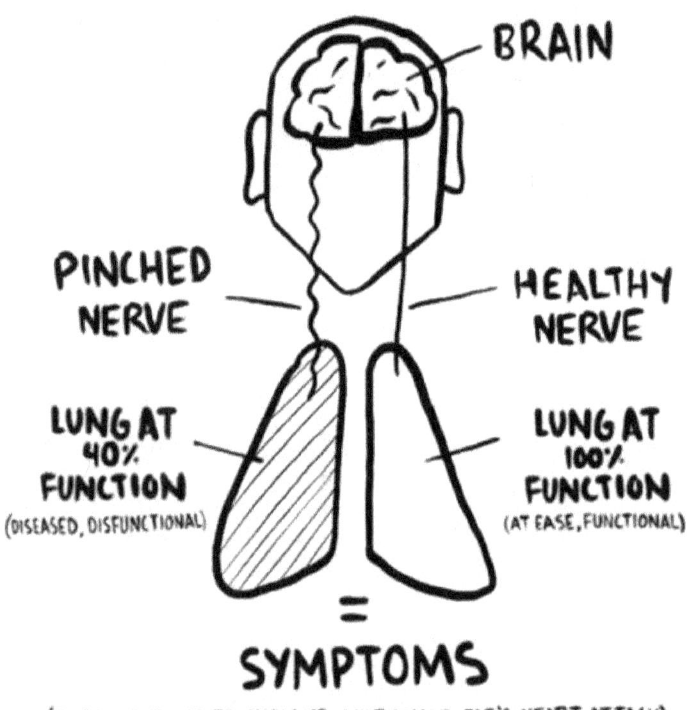


*Picture 12: Brain-Body Diagram*

"Get to the source of the problem! Fix the subluxation and restore proper nerve function so the body can do what it does best: heal!"

"Remember B.J. Palmer's words: 'The body heals from above down, inside-out!'"

"Before we end for today, I want to mention some miraculous changes that occurred in my body after receiving chiropractic for the last five years. Ever since I fell from the tree so many years ago – and I must say, it took a bit for me to put two and two together – I developed asthma and pretty bad allergies. I seemed to catch every seasonal cold, had constant sinusitis with a persistent cough, and also had a pretty severe case of dyslexia (or ADD, if you wish). Although I was diagnosed with dyslexia in first grade, in retrospect, it is easy to understand that the pain-killing drugs – whether provided by Big Pharma or the drug dealer in the local park – only furthered my inability to read and comprehend. But prior to the fall causing a compression fracture of the bottom vertebra in my back L5, I had not yet suffered any asthma or allergy symptoms in my life. I now understand that an impact strong enough to fracture a vertebra in my back could easily have caused other damage to different areas of the spine with maybe more subtle, insidious onsets of symptoms. After being under chiropractic care for several years, I can tell you that those other symptoms, such as asthma and allergies, just disappeared. What's more, I have not been sick in many years. What other nerve disruptions were corrected, and what other disease processes were helped? I guess I will never know. But I'm glad they are handled!"

Joey seemed to be contemplating something, then cleared his throat.

"You all have done so well. I'm proud of you all. The next bit of information is quite a lot and very important. It's too late in the day to go into it, so I say we all get in the car and drive down the coast to the Big Sur Inn. They have an amazing organic menu there. Let's go celebrate!"

There was no argument among us. As much as we wanted more, we also knew we were filled up for the day.

It was a beautiful day in Carmel, and as we drove down the coast highway, I think all of us were feeling grateful, grateful to Joey, and grateful for each other's support and growing friendship.

I should mention that while Alice grabbed a shotgun, Judy and I were content holding hands and rubbing elbows.

## Mental / Emotional / Spiritual Stressors

I must say, it was a struggle being on my own for a week. Trying to stick to the diet wasn't easy, and I admit I did cheat a bit. And, for some reason, I had a hard time not thinking about Judy. Nevertheless, I was committed, and when I arrived at Judy's house at about 5:30 p.m. on Friday, I was just in time for a nice dinner. It was, of course, keto-friendly: baked wild salmon and sweet potato and romaine salad with avocado, pecans, and blueberries dressed with red wine vinegar and avocado oil. It was amazing!

As I awoke early Saturday morning, I felt more energy than I had in years, and my mind seemed to be moving a mile a minute. So much happened in the last few days. My right leg, which was minus the foot, was healing quicker than expected. I saw the doc yesterday afternoon, and as he was examining the area, he commented that he was happy with what he saw. He said he didn't usually see this type of procedure heal so fast. He also commented on the fact that I had lost 18 pounds since I was released from the hospital. I hadn't even thought about it, although Joey did weigh us in on Day 1. I started at 264 and was now at 246 – pretty good!

He was happy and said that he was sure that the pre-scribed diabetic-related diet was helping. *I had to bite my tongue before I spilled the beans about my new health coach, Joey, and how he was starving me to death*, I thought with a silent chuckle.

When I got to the kitchen, I realized I was the first one up. I saw the keto meter sitting on the counter, so I took my readings. To my surprise, my ketones were at 1.0! Joey would approve. My glucose was still high at 154 but was still down from the 190 range it tended to stay in, even with the drugs I used to take for it.

I was just sipping my coffee when Joey made his way into the kitchen. I bid him good morning and then men-tioned my numbers. He was pleased and said that I was getting younger every day!

I laughed and said rhetorically, "That would be great if I actually could get my youth back."

As I looked Joey in the eye, he said, "That is exactly what we are going to do, Fred - *turn back your biological clock.* You'll be younger by the time we're done with this process." Then he added, "If you are going to continue to court my mom – and you do have my permission – I want to make sure you are not only around for the duration, but that you are healthy too."

I could see that Joey saw the doubt in my eyes, so he decided to fill in the blanks. About that time, my beautiful new girlfriend came down the stairs. She looked prettier every time I saw her, and I told her so on the stoop.

This Saturday morning marked our fourth week of class. Joey was already set up, and everyone was in the kitchen drinking their keto coffee and visiting. I offered Judy a cup and proceeded to prepare the whipped cream before dripping the coffee. This ritual became such a favorite part of my day. I never would have guessed that coffee could taste so good.

# 24-Hour Fast

Joey was excited about my testing results and said that was a perfect way to start this week's class. He said that today, we would expand our fasting window to a twenty-four-hour fast. We all ate last night at about 6:00 p.m., and we would make today a fast day. It meant we would not have our next meal until 6:00 p.m. tonight.

This would drive us even more into ketosis and get the body reaching deep down into the fat stores. It was how we became "metabolically flexible" - when our body can easily switch between the two fuels, glucose and ketones. Joey said this is what we want to accomplish: metabolic flexibility.

He said that coffee was available and we could consume coffee and whipping cream, MTC oil, ghee, or whatever suited us. As long as we were just consuming oils, we would be feeding ketosis and not spiking insulin. This was going to help our body become a better fat burner. He said that if, for any reason, during the twenty-four-hour fast, we didn't feel like continuing and needed to eat, go ahead. Sometimes, your body needs to work up to it, and we had plenty of time to convert to fat burning. He mentioned that we had the rest of our lives to get healthy.

Next, Joey got started on the lesson for the day. He began by giving a short recap of how physical stressors affected our health, then said that we were going to cover the other two stressors – mental/ emotional/ spiritual stressors.

"Okay," Joey said, "let's get started!"

"Take this as you will," Joey started, "but do you remember when I drew the three-legged stool, then I added 'innate intelligence' in the guise of a smiley face on top? It became obvious to me that this innate intelligence is not given enough credit in the world of Western medicine. Even though the third side of the health triangle represents mental/ emotional health, I believe the spiritual element or innate intelligence is grossly underestimated."

"I'm not going to get up on a soap box here, but I believe that for anything to happen regarding us and our lives, a decision comes first. How did Shakespeare say it? 'To be or not to be' – I believe that still is the question. So, even though we are now going to discuss how the emotional side of the health pyramid affects our health, we must also look to who is making the decisions about what, when, and how. You know that statement, 'If it's to be, it's up to me?' Well, I agree. I'm not going to go much farther on this line right now, as the purpose of our meeting is to help you handle your current state of health based on the most current understanding and discoveries in the field of natural healing."

As Joey walked to the table and took a sip from his water bottle, I looked inward. I was astonished at how little attention I ever really gave as to who I really was and what motivated me. As so much of this information was new and fresh, I just let Joey lead onward. This was turning into an adventure, and I liked the feel of it. Something inside me was igniting and gave me a surge of energy, but it was different from what I remember feeling in a long time, if ever. I was ready to change and prepared for the world.

After a few moments, Joey walked over to the white-board and wrote, "What your mind is doing to your body." I could feel a well of emotion build up inside me. He really didn't have to explain much, but I was amazed how just a few words could throw me onto a mental rollercoaster. Right then, the loss of my dear wife, the alienation from my kids, and my failing health hit me like a ton of bricks.

I suddenly felt that empty feeling I got so often that made me want to indulge in alcohol, ice cream, or eat whatever there was in the cupboard. I suddenly felt tired and sad. I looked at my breakfast, which was a cup of organic shade-grown coffee with organic whipping cream in it, and thought to myself, *I'll never make it.* I must say that I came moments away from deciding to pack up my things, head to the nearest liquor store, buy myself a gallon of cheap gin, and sail off into the sunset. And I almost did.

Judy sensed what was up, slid her chair closer to me, and put her hand on mine. I didn't even realize how tightly I was gripping the arm of the chair. But when I felt her warm, soft, loving hand touch mine, a wave of tension seemed just to evaporate. Then, for the first time in years, I felt loved. Joey came over and put his hand on my shoulder, saying nothing but knowing all. Even Alice seemed moved; I could see it in her eyes. These guys cared, and for the second time in the last few days, I had hope.

"We're all glad you're here, Fred," Joey started. "You have suffered more than your fair share of losses. I want to let you know that you are safe here. You don't have to hide your emotions; we are all here to support each other. Are you okay with that?"

Judy's gentle squeeze of my hand ensured me that I was okay and in the right place. For the first time since the death of my dear wife, I cried. After a minute, I composed myself. I could feel the calmness of Judy's touch unwavering through my emotions. I felt a bit of embarrassment but, at the same time, a tremendous amount of relief.

"Thank you," was all I could muster at first. Then, after some time, I addressed the group – my group, my new family. "Joey, thank you so much for caring and taking time out of your life to help me. When I first woke up in that hospital bed, minus my leg, I thought my life was over, and I really didn't care. I was alone – my family was gone or had distanced themselves from me. For a moment, I lost all hope. But then, after awakening from a drug-induced night's sleep, I heard the bantering and arguing of your sister and mother on the other side of the dividing curtain. I must say, Alice, that through it all and as unpleasant as it seemed, it was apparent how much you love your mother. I was envious of both of you. I'm not even sure if any of my kids know where I am. I left a message for my daughter to call me before I was admitted to the hospital, but as of today, I still have not heard back from her."

"I think that mentally and emotionally – even spiritually – I gave up. So, if you suggest that my thoughts could affect my health, I think you made your point simply by writing those words on the board. Thank you so much, but what can I do? How do I fix this?"

"That's a great question, and thanks for asking," Joey replied. "This is a big subject; we can discuss it in more detail later. But I want to bring up a couple of thoughts and suggestions. In fact, let's do this now."

"For now, I want to go over a few things that I incorporated into my life and daily routine that help me stay on track. Some of it comes from Dr. McCollum, and others from friends and mentors I have met on my own journey."

"First off, Dr. McCollum taught me several phrases that finally kicked in and became part of my thought process."

"The first thing he taught me was, *'What you think about, you talk about; what you talk about, you bring about.'* He told me this over and over and over again until, one day, I caught myself obsessively dwelling on something I did not want to have happen. I worried about it for what seemed like days. Finally, after a terrible night's sleep of not sleeping, I found out that my worst dreams had come true. I brought into existence exactly what I was thinking about, and it almost killed me. The stress of the situation, which I will spare you the details of, had such an impact on me that my old lower back injury flared up so badly I could barely get out of bed. I could not think of anything I had done physically to bring it about. That is when I called Dr. McCollum. I was so happy to hear his wife Patty's angelic voice assure me that I would be alright and that I should get myself down to the office as soon as I could."

"Of course, Dr. McCollum had me on my feet in now time. He understood my body so well. He explained what I already knew, that L5 had slipped again. I was amazed at how quickly that adjustment worked."

"Then Dr. McCollum asked what I did and how I had pulled my back out this time. That is when it hit me. 'Doc,' I said, 'I've been worrying about something all week. I've been obsessed and afraid of the outcome. You know what, doc? I brought this on with my stinkin-thinkin!'"

"So, I learned the hard way. What you think about, you talk about, and what you talk about, you bring about. That is when I consciously started to practice focusing on the things I wanted, appreciated, or found pleasing. This has been a process, but it grows on you. And you know what? I find it works."

"Number two, he told me repeatedly, '*99.99% of the things you worry about never happen.*' Again, it took me months, if not years, to realize the truth of that statement. And just think of all the stress hormones released when you worry. Remember, those stress hormones can become inflammatory over time. So far, Dr. McCollum has been right; nothing has killed me yet!"

"Number three. Remember I told you I had a chance to attend a Live It To Lead It seminar that Dr. McCollum invited me to? Well, there was this speaker named Ben Azadi. In part of his talk, he kept eluding to this newly discovered vitamin. He said that it had magic powers that could dramatically change your health. He called it vitamin G. He continued to tell us about the magical characteristics of this vitamin. Then he let the cat out of the bag. Vitamin G stood for 'Gratitude."

"Be grateful," he said, "once you stop focusing on all the bad stuff that is going on in your life and find things and people and situations to be grateful for, your life will change."

"He explained that our emotional responses cause various chemicals called neurotransmitters to be released in our body. Serotonin and dopamine are the two critical 'feel good' neurotransmitters. By exercising gratitude or being grateful, you can change your emotional state."

"Number four - your morning ritual. Get yourself a journal and start writing everything you want to see happen. Only I want you to write it as if it were that way right now, in the present moment. You can write about how good it feels to be healthy, how rewarding it is to help people, how stabilizing it is to have no debt, plenty of savings, and a great income source, how much you love your family, how well they are doing, how much you love to spend time with them, how proud you are of them; how happy you are with your present love interest; and how much fun you have together."

Joey paused, looked at us, and said, "You see how this goes? It may not all come to fruition at once, but as you continue to do this every day, your life will change because you are willing it to change."

At that point, Joey reached into his briefcase and pulled out several notebooks. He walked over and handed one to each of us, including Alice, who seemed happy to receive it.

"Okay," Joey said, "here is the exercise I want you to do every day, every morning. Take a pen and start writing. Go ahead – I want you to do this right now."

Joey passed out a sheet of paper with a list of questions to help us write out some goals. He said that it may seem difficult at first and that he would give us twenty minutes to get it done. Of course, he noted that these techniques took practice, just like learning to play a musical instrument or some new coordinated skill. He said that if we kept it up long enough, miracles would happen.

I believed him.

Looking at the list, I realized I had not given many of these subjects the time of day for many years, if not ever.

At the top of the paper were simple directions.

Write out a thought regarding each of the following subjects. Write them in the present time, as though they are happening right now in your life. See if you can get the senses to go along with each. For instance, the smell of the air, the climate, the position of your body, and the emotions accompanying each. The more detailed you can imagine, the better - you dare to dream. Repeat this exercise every day and modify your visions as you desire. Here are some examples, but you can get creative as you go along.

- How do you see your health and your physical activity?
- How is your family/ love relationship doing?
- How is your work and your professional life?
- What does your financial situation look like?
- What hobbies, sports, traveling, etc., would you like to do?

Joey interjected, "This exercise may seem tough initially; it was for me. But the more you do it, the better it gets and the more the good things come true in your life."

"I recommend doing this for ninety days. Only do those that you feel comfortable with. If you feel this exercise has been helpful at the end of ninety days, then continue at will."

"Go ahead and start. You have twenty minutes."

After twenty minutes, he restarted us by saying, "Okay, so for your homework, I would like you to spend ten to twenty minutes each morning writing out how you see your life. This is a great process to help you keep on track and reduce some of the mental stress we seem to put on ourselves."

At that, we took a twenty-minute bathroom break.

## Chemical Stressors

"Next, we will talk about the chemical stressors affecting our health." He said this is a big subject and that once we understand it, we can't help but make better decisions regarding our health and lifestyle."

"We are now going to explore what is probably the biggest cause of chronic inflammation in your body and what to do about it. Remember the statement by Dr. Dan Pompa? 'Fix the cell to get well?' Well, today, you will understand what this means."

"But before we delve into this concept, I want to say a few more words about stress and how it affects both your body and your mind. There is this thing called the 'fight or flight' mechanism – I'm sure you have heard about it. We must acquire a good working understanding of this now because it is really at the core of your health, well-being, and ability to survive. Functioning correctly, it will keep you alive. Unfortunately, in today's world, too many people are stuck in a fight or flight mode, causing the stress hormone cortisone to be constantly secreted by the adrenal glands. This chronic cortisol causes chronic inflammation, among other things, but the inflammation alone is responsible for so many health issues. By the way, practicing the techniques we just went over can go a long way in shutting off this 'fight or flight' mechanism."

## Autonomic nervous system

"So, let me start with a brief explanation of something called the autonomic nervous system. It's basically a part of the nervous system that works automatically or unconsciously and influences our internal organs – you know, keeping our heart beating, our lungs working, and our gut digesting and eliminating, as well as influencing sexual arousal. You don't have to think about it; it keeps on. "Well," Joey paused, "sexual arousal may be the exception." This caused a giggle from Judy. Slightly embarrassed, I remained quiet."

"The autonomic nervous system," Joey continued, "is divided into two parts, the sympathetic and parasympathetic systems. Without getting too involved here, the parasympathetic nervous system can be considered the 'rest and digest' system. In contrast, the sympathetic nervous system can be considered the 'fight or flight' system.

"Today, we will focus on the sympathetic 'fight or flight' system so we can better understand how acute or chronic stress impacts our health. Interestingly enough, this system is chemically driven, albeit driven by chemicals that our body makes."

"Here's how the sympathetic nervous system works. Any time we are threatened with a loss of survival, whether real or imagined, a stimulus-response mechanism goes into play to help ensure survival. For example, when you burn your hand on a stove, your reflexes prompt you to pull it away. If you smell smoke or something caustic, your first response could be fear with a heightened heartbeat. Then, you might hold your breath and seek fresh air. If you are driving a car and need to swerve quickly to avoid an accident, you startle, snap back into the present time, and acutely take in the environment and any perceived danger in it. If someone or something threatens you or your loved ones verbally or even physically, you rise to the occasion by either fighting, fleeing, or potentially using reason to settle the situation."

"In all these cases, a chemical response occurs in your body through the endocrine or hormone systems. Your brain perceives the danger through any or all of your senses. It transfers the data to the endocrine or hormone system, which begins at the hypothalamus and pituitary glands in your brain. These glands secrete chemicals into your bloodstream, which travel to targeted endocrine or hormone-secreting organs in your body to trigger a response. And it all happens in a nanosecond."

"So, basically, your nerves send electrical messages to your brain targeting something called the 'master gland' or hypothalamus gland located in the center of your brain. This, in turn, now sends chemical or electrical messengers down to the pituitary gland, which sits right below the hypothalamus. The pituitary gland then squirts chemical hormones into the bloodstream. These hormones reach targeted endocrine glands through the blood and deliver a message, which tells that gland to squirt different hormones into the bloodstream that travel to hormone receptor sites located on the cell walls in different organs so that the message can be received and acted upon by the cells. Whew! Bodies are pretty amazing! It works kind of like the postal service; each message or letter has a particular address on it. These specific messages are directed to different addresses or, in the case of your hormones, to specific cells, organs, or other glands where the messages are read. Then the actions are carried out."

"Just to help with any confusion: endocrine glands are things like your thyroid, parathyroid, thymus, pancreas, adrenals, and testes. These all respond to hormone messengers they receive from the pituitary gland."

# ENDOCRINE SYSTEM

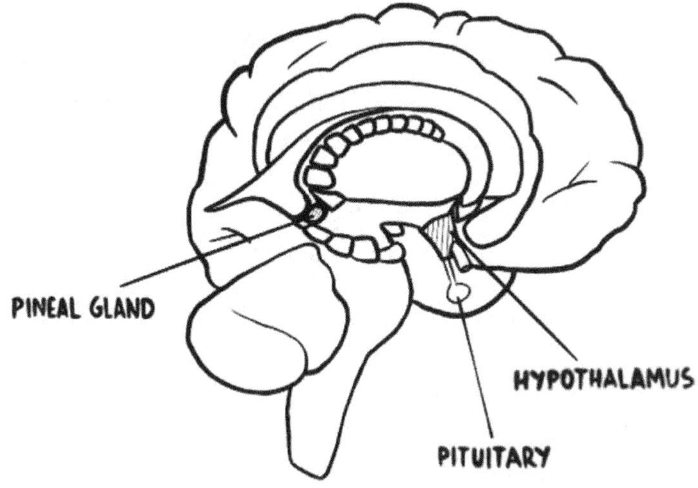


*Picture 13: Endocrine or Hormone Control Center*

"All right, let's get back to the 'fight or flight' part of the endocrine system, which is part of the sympathetic nervous system."

"Your adrenal glands are the main pair of glands targeted in this 'fight or flight' response. 'Adrenal' literally translates to 'on top of kidneys.' They are almond-sized glands that produce a huge amount of different hormones. In the case of 'fight or flight,' they produce the hormones adrenaline and norepinephrine. These increase your heart and respirator rate, pushing blood and oxygen to your muscles for 'fight or flight' while, at the same time, constricting the blood vessels going to systems like your immune system, digestive system, and brain. This allows for superhuman strength at a primordial survival level so that your survival instinct can better react to the perceived emergency. Have you ever heard of a mom picking up a car to get her child out from under it? There are many examples of how the adrenal glands and this superhuman strength thing work."

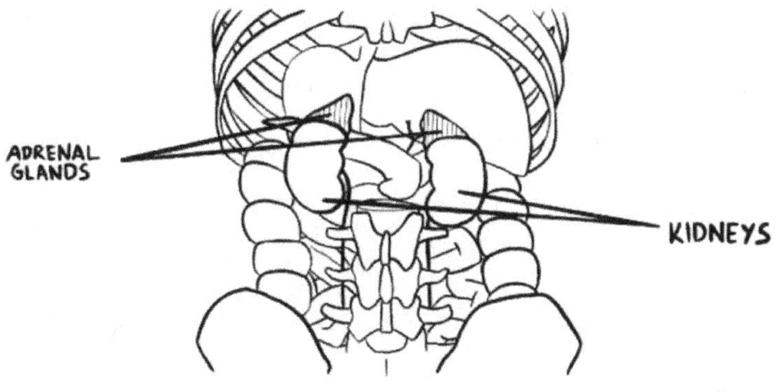


*Picture 14: Adrenal Glands*

"Once the emergency is over, the autonomic nervous system is supposed to balance back out for everyday operation. The sympathetic 'fight or flight' and the parasympathetic 'rest and digest' systems ebb and flow appropriately."

"Herein lies the problem. Today, we are faced with a tremendous amount of stress, real or imagined. Not only is the media filled with constant negative news, but people are also faced with threats to survival from everything from financial burdens, family breakups, political unrest, planetary disasters, and – of course, the main reason I am telling you all this – the terrible state and continuing decline of health in our country. Again, we are rated forty-seventh in the world for health."

"Acute stress has immediate effects, and our bodies have been programed to respond to this throughout eternity. But the chronic stress that so many people are under today is creating a myriad of tremendous, life-threatening health conditions. Chronic stress, by definition, tells us that we have a chronically lower immune response, a chronically lower digestive function, and even a chronically lower mental-emotional tone. Many who are suffering from chronic stress are living in fear and experiencing chronic anxiety, depression, and other devastating and even debilitating emotions."

"One of the big problems with chronic stress – be it physical, chemical, emotional, or a combination of all three – is that many vitally important systems in our bodies are chronically shut down. It causes a breakdown of our organs and a buildup of toxins as our digestive and elimination systems are not working well. We now have millions of Americans suffering from the consequences of something called leaky gut syndrome, where the intestinal walls become inflamed. This inflammation opens up spaces between the intestinal cell walls, allowing unhealthy particles to move across our intestinal walls, transporting toxins and even undigested food particles and even unwanted microbes from the colon into the blood stream and then to the actual cells and organs in our body. It causes inflammation at a cellular level and is at the heart of the beginning of autoimmune disease. Autoimmune means the body starts attacking itself. This, by the way, includes inflammation, toxification, and premature aging or degeneration of the brain."

"And this, my friends, is one major reason our bodies become toxic and then diseased. When this chronic inflammation remains in and around our cells and organs, accumulated toxins inside the cells turn on bad genes. This can trigger the expression of those bad genes, resulting in chronic disease."

"So, now you may have a better understanding of how chronic disease is caused by chronic inflammation and that chronic inflammation is caused by toxins. Yes?"

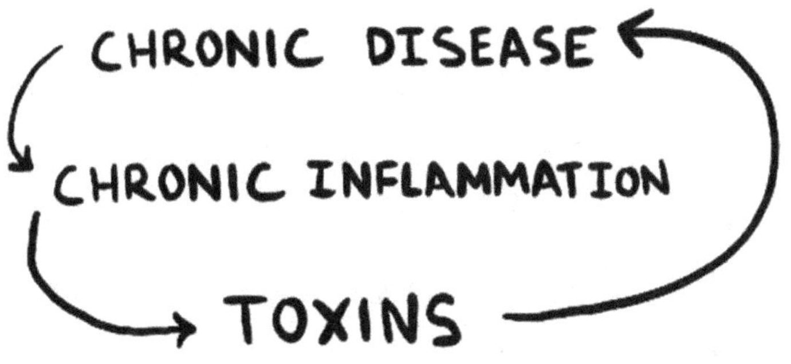


*Picture 15*

"Now, it is important to understand that we are surrounded by an ever-growing world of toxicity. Since the Industrial Revolution, over 87,000 chemicals and industrial byproducts have been dumped into our air, water, and soil. Many of these substances combined create yet even more different and toxic substances. More and more radioactive and electromagnetic exposure only add to the fray."

"Now, we are hearing about 'forever chemical' which won't break down in the environment. These are PFAS or 'polyfluoroalkyl substances. These are a class of about 10,000 chemicals with non-stick and detergent properties now found in our waterways and soil. Of course, these PFAS chemicals have been associated with everything from cancer, thyroid disease to kidney disease and autoimmune disease."

"Sorry to paint such a gloomy picture, but I must add that our soils have been systematically depleted of minerals and other nutrients due to the large commercial farm industry and their lack of understanding of sustainable farming, let alone their usage of toxic herbicides, pesticides, and commercial chemical fertilizers."

"Okay, so we live in an ever-increasing toxic environment, whether from our own body's byproducts or from the polluted planet. All of these can have a dramatic effect on our health. The more susceptible each of our bodies are genetically (meaning that when bad genes turn on, so do bad diseases), the more likely our exposure to these toxins will result in chronic disease."

"So, since we can't magically clean up the whole world's toxic load, the next best option is to get our immune system as strong as possible while working to eliminate as much of the toxic buildup in our bodies as possible. It may seem ominous, but it is doable and rewarding."

"So again, how do you handle chronic disease? Of course, remove the toxins from your environment and from your body and then repair any damage done to all the systems and organs of the body. This needs to be addressed, and as Dr. Pompa has explained so well, all the way down to the cellular level. The good news is, there is hope; something can be done about it."

"This starts by consuming only healthy oils and eating only organically grown foods. Of course, this means staying away from all commercially grown and GMO foods which, if not eliminated, would sabotage any attempts to repair or correct the cellular damage done."

"This is the subject we will be working on for the next several weeks. It is going to be exciting to watch the transformation of your body. In fact, today, I want us all to get pictures of our faces and profiles; it's fun to watch the transformation."

"Let's take a break, and when we come back, I'm going to have you watch a three-minute video by Dr. Bruce Lipton. I mentioned him already. This video will really emphasize the concept of how toxins affect the cell's health and drive home the concept of fixing the cell to get well."

*Video can be found at:*

*(I highly recommend you readers to watch this video)*

Now, I'm not much of a scientist, but the video Joey just played for us made a lot of sense to me and, again, had me on the edge of my seat. What this guy Bruce Lipton was saying was that my current health condition is a reflection of the unhealthy choices I made along the way, coupled with the toxic environment I lived in and was exposed to. But he also alluded to the fact that if I change my environment – in this case, what I put into my body – while eliminating the acquired and stored toxins out of my body, I could change the future of my health. Humm!

Basically, what Dr. Lipton was saying was that the cell (and its wall) is probably the most intelligent part of life. It constantly reads the environment and adapts. He likened the cell wall to a computer chip. In his words, it is "a liquid crystal semiconductor with gates and channels with a read/write mechanism." He was basically saying that each cell in our body, being alive, is like a minicomputer that can think for itself. Each cell, having once been a stem cell and converting to the particular cell it became – a liver, kidney, heart, or finger cell – has its own program to follow. Still, it will read the environment and adapt. Each cell is even programmed to last a certain length of time and then self-destruct. I remember Joey mentioned before the term called *apoptosis,* or "programmed cell death." What happens to the cells and these programs when confronted with the three causes of stress, especially the chemical one, is that they either mutate into bad cells, become senile and useless, cause disease, or die prematurely.

What struck me most was the part about how if you put a bunch of live cells in a toxic environment, they would start to get sick and die, but if you took them out of that dirty environment and put them in a healthy one, they would immediately start to become healthier and live.

This was pretty amazing. So that is how the "Fix the Cell to Get Well" thing this Dr. Dan Pompa talks about fits into the equation. I was actually starting to get this stuff.

The funny thing was that I wanted to be mad at somebody and blame someone, but all I could do at that moment was look inward. What was happening? I was feeling warm; I could feel my heart beating like it was trying to get out of my chest, and I felt like I was gasping for air. I felt like screaming, 'I want to live'.

I looked at Judy, who was deep in her thoughts, then asked the question.

"Joey, what can we do? How do we get our health back?"

Even Alice was quiet; I think Joey was beginning to win her over.

"First of all," Joey started, "I want to go over what Dr. Lipton was saying. It is important to understand what is happening in the cells of our body that is making us sick. We can no longer walk into a doctor's office and drop the body off to get fixed like we would taking our car to the auto shop. We need to be the ones making the decisions regarding what should happen."

"So, Dr. Lipton was saying that these cell walls allow things in and out of the cells. They are liquid crystal semiconductors with gates and channels. When they are in a healthy environment, they work; when exposed to toxic environments, they get sick."

"The cells are life, right?"

"So, this is where Dr. Dan Pompa's simple phrase 'fix the cell to get well' comes in. And that is the magic. If we can change the environment – not only around where we live but also the environment around the cells – we can get well."

"Let's look at it. Toxins are produced in our cells as we burn fuel, such as glucose or ketones (fat), for energy. Any fuel being burned has a byproduct, just like the exhaust that comes out of your car. This, as we know, is usually toxic. This is true in the cell as well. So, those gates and channels Dr. Lipton was talking about are designed to eliminate toxins from the cells. They also allow fuel into the cells. In fact, as he said, the cells read the environment and adapt. Hormones, vitamins, minerals, and many other substances also act in and communicate with the cells. The cell membrane acts as the gatekeeper, ensuring that only good stuff gets through and bad stuff gets out – at least until toxins enter the equation. That is when inflammation can occur, and if the body's systems can't correct this, a disease state can begin."

"Now, the body was designed to survive through all sorts of adverse circumstances. And it has done pretty well over the eons. The problems are several. For one, man has created some 80,000 chemicals in the last couple hundred years. Most of them are harmful, carcinogenic, neurotoxic, or just plain deadly. The powers that be, such as the CDC,

FDA, and NIH, turned the other cheek, you might say, allowing these to be dumped into our food, water, air, and even into the clothes we wear. Most of us have more than one environmental waste dump in our homes. Just look under your sink, your medicine cabinet, or the garage. They are filled with what Dr. Lipton was talking about – the *adverse environment,* I think he calls it."

"Our bodies are built to last. They are self-sustaining organisms designed to survive. They do well, especially when they are challenged. They like diversity and thrive to survive under the wildest conditions, hormesis. But our poor liver, our major detoxification organ, was not designed with the understanding that so many toxic substances would ever be created. The food we eat is processed, altered, and bastardized. Pharmaceuticals, sugar, and white processed flour – now mostly genetically modified (GMO) – were pushed on us. Eventually, depending on many factors, our body loses the ability to detoxify all this stuff, kind of like a clogged oil filter in your car or a clogged filter on a vacuum cleaner. It stops working, and toxins build up in our bodies. These toxins damage the cells, block the gates and channels, and even eat away the cell wall. This lowers our resistance to the environment, causing a weakened immune system and weakened cellular response."

"All of these toxins culminate in one thing: cellular inflammation. When this becomes chronic, we become ill. Left unchecked, we end up dying of some terrible disease. No one dies of 'old age' anymore. What causes chronic disease? Chronic inflammation. What causes chronic inflammation? Toxins."

Joey stopped talking for a minute and, taking a big breath, looked each of us in the eye. I believe what he saw gave him hope. We were stunned, transfixed in our own thoughts.

"Okay, you all," Joey said, "guess what? It's 5:30 p.m.! You just finished a twenty-four-hour fast. Congratulations! That is it for today. Let's eat!"

Boy, I could hardly believe it. The day had gone by so quickly that I wasn't even hungry. When I mentioned it to Joey, he said that my body was doing really well at fat adapting. We checked my ketones and found that they were at 2.5, which Joey said was a great range. Both Judy and Alice were also in ketosis. They, too, did not feel hungry all day. This was getting fun!

We had an amazing meal, as usual. This cellular healing lifestyle was growing on me.

Joey preset the oven to start a few hours earlier and had a beef brisket cooking on low heat. It smelled amazing. When he pulled it out of the oven, the aroma almost knocked me over. I could see yellow onions and various zucchini in the pot, stewing along with the beef.

Judy's kitchen was pretty well set up. I didn't realize there were two ovens until Joey opened the second one and removed a tray of roasted vegetables. There were carrots, red onions, some yellow and green squash, and red bell peppers. The cloves of roasted garlic mixed with the rosemary well.

We enjoyed some of the most tender beef I've ever had, smothered in its own juices. The veggies were just right, not overcooked; again, I could use all the butter I wanted.

Later, we all gathered in the living room and watched a couple of old movies. It was so comfortable, leaving me missing my family again.

# CHAPTER 7

# You Are What You Ate!

I woke up Sunday morning to the smell of bacon cooking. I thought I must be dreaming and lay in bed for a minute, making sure I was awake. Once I was certain I was awake and that it actually was bacon I was smelling, I decided that I better go investigate.

After putting myself together, I made my way into the kitchen, now using one crutch. I was surprised to see Joey at the stove with a chef hat on.

"Good morning," he said without so much of a hint of recognition that I was confused.

"What are you doing, Joey?" I asked sincerely.

"What does it look like? I'm cooking bacon."

"I can see that. I'm not blind, and I can still smell. But I don't get it. What happened to the starvation diet?"

He laughed and said, "Today –" He was interrupted by his mom's voice.

Judy was just making her way down the stairs, and I lost all consciousness, at least regarding food. She looked gorgeous this morning, and I swore she looked twenty years younger than when I met her in the hospital. I said as much, and I could see her face flush as I did so. How did I get so lucky? I wondered to myself.

"Good morning, Fred. You look handsome today yourself," Judy said.

I felt pleased. Even though I wanted to find out what it was that smelled like bacon, I made sure to freshen up before I made my way into the kitchen. So, I pulled a fresh shirt from the closet – I had a few I brought with me. I felt good this morning, full of energy, and when I saw Judy, I actually felt a bit of excitement in my groin. A stir of testosterone, perhaps. I hadn't really felt that for years.

"What are you cooking, Joey?" Judy said as though she suddenly noticed him and the wonderful smell for the first time.

"Bacon," he retorted. "What's with you two? Haven't you ever eaten bacon before?"

His comment seemed to fall on deaf ears because Judy and I were in a deep conversation about the orchids I had delivered yesterday and how much they brought out the color of her skin. She was giggling and telling me that I was being silly but that she loved orchids and was surprised to receive them. They were delivered about the time we stopped class for the day. I was recalling how happy she was and that she and I walked into her garden to enjoy some time with ourselves. I reminisced on how nice it was to sit on her little cement bench nestled among the primroses and cyclamen, which grew under a beautifully trimmed oak tree. We talked about many things. She started to ask about my family, and could see the sadness in my eyes. She said she understood. She paused for a moment, then mentioned that maybe someday, she and I could go visit them. The tears came silently down my cheeks. She reached up and touched them with her hand. After a moment, she said, "Fred, you are such a sweet man. I am so happy to have met you."

Alice's voice once again disrupted my reverie. "Good morning, all. What smells so good?" she asked no one in particular.

"Bacon," we all said at once with a little volume added.

Judy, Joey, and I all looked at each other and burst out laughing hysterically.

"What's so funny?" she asked somewhat defensively.

That only made us laugh harder. I had to find a chair and sit down before falling off my one good leg.

When we finally settled down and had explained to Alice why her question was met with such a reaction, almost simultaneously, we three looked at Joey and said, "What's with bacon anyway?" which sent all of us into another fit of laughter.

"What's going on?" I finally managed to ask Joey between explosive giggles.

"Hormones," Joey replied. "Your bodies are starting to work again. By changing the foods you've been eating and varying how much and when you eat them, we are 'bio-hacking' your endocrine system into working again."

"You see, we've been forcing your bodies to stop the old paradigm of constantly snacking on or feasting on crappy foods that require all the energy you can muster to digest. We've also eliminated many inflammatory foods, so your physiology is changing. In other words, you have a different body today than you had just a few weeks ago."

"Fred, you actually look years younger already. The swelling is gone under your eyes, and your whole body looks fitter."

"He's right," Alice piped in. "I've been noticing that myself. I would have never imagined that just changing foods could make such a difference. I just weighed myself this morning, and I have lost 5 pounds. This is amazing. I've been trying to get below 140 for years, and today, I weighed in at 138!"

"Yessssss!" we all yelled.

"So, what's with the bacon?" I asked again as I felt my stomach growling. I couldn't believe that he was going to feed us an actual breakfast.

"Today is a *feast day*. Today, we get to eat all day!"

"What?" we all exclaimed in unison.

Joey began to explain. "Our bodies love change. Change challenges our body and makes all the systems we have come into play. Imagine once being an athlete but then spending ten years sitting at a desk, never exercising. Then, one day, an old buddy comes to town and says, 'Come on, Fred, let's go hit some balls.' The next thing you know, you're out there on the court playing tennis with your old college roommate in the heat of battle. You are likely to either pull a muscle or be sore as hell the next day. It's a bit too steep of a gradient. You'd have been better off working your body up to the challenge."

"Well, that is what we've been doing with *diet variation.* You see, Dr Dan Pompa really mastered this thing. By engaging in feast and famine cycles, we are actually biohacking our endocrine system to start working again on all cylinders. Today, we will eat three keto meals. This ensures your body doesn't think it is starving, so it will continue to shed weight! Let's eat!"

Since we were all so engaged in conversation – and quite honestly, since I was focusing all my attention on Judy – we didn't pay attention to what Joey was cooking. When he brought over the most beautiful stir-fry omelet I ever saw, I must have gasped for air because everyone looked at me at once. I reflected that we were restricted to just two meals for the last several days. I decided this was a fun and always surprising way to get healthier.

I laughed and said, "I never thought I'd be so happy to see food. I just took for granted that it would always be there. Not eating has been such a challenge."

I thought about my words as I heaped a huge portion of food on my plate. I was a bit dismayed that Joey had not provided biscuits and gravy, or at least toast. I said as much. It was, of course, met with a giggle from Judy as her foot reached out to find the only one I had left. When she touched me, I was filled with goosebumps.

**Biohacking**

As we started to eat, Joey began to explain ***biohacking*** via ***intermittent fasting***, the ***ketogenic diet***, along with the added benefits of ***diet variation***, and something called ***ancient healing strategies***, which would not only help reduce inflammation in our body but also help us burn our own stored fat. As a result of these *biohacks*, we would begin to detoxify our body at a cellular level. He said this created an environment where our cell walls could heal and become more permeable or biologically and metabolically flexible. He reminded us of what Dr. Bruce Lipton said about cells in a favorable environment immediately starting to get well and thrive. "So," Joey continued, "in just these last few days, your bodies are actually reading the environment better and more able to absorb the hormones that attach to the receptor sites on the cell."

He said the cleaner the internal environment, the fewer hormones needed to get the job done. Then he asked a great question.

"If you had the choice of allowing your body to be toxic and inflamed by the myriad of chemicals, heavy metals, molds, and unfriendly opportunist bugs, we accumulated all these years – which meant dumping gobs of synthetic or animal hormones into your bodies in the hopes that they could find their way to an available unclogged cell receptor – or, you had the chance to clean up your body's environment, repair the cells, organs, tissue, and even your brain by removing inflammation, learn how not to re-pollute it, restore proper nutrition, and promote proper nerve and hormone function, which would you choose?"

Wow – the million-dollar question. I felt so lucky to meet this family. I was getting more excited about my future every second of every day.

I wondered what would have happened if I learned this information earlier. Would I have changed, or would I have still waited until it was almost too late, continuing to eat, drink, and be merry all the way to my grave? Something was beginning to stir in me; I felt motivated. I wanted to get myself as healthy as I could and then go tell the world about what happened. People needed to get this information before it was too late.

I said out loud and to no one in particular, "This is so amazing! I want to tell my family, my friends – anyone who will listen. Thank you. I think I just found my new purpose in life.

I looked at Judy and could see the tears in her eyes. Even Alice was resolute. She shook her head and said, "This is amazing information, Joey. Thank you for allowing me, your big sister, to be a part of this. I think you just saved me from a miserable life. I didn't say anything before, but at my last doctor check-up, she told me I was pre-diabetic. I didn't want to hear it, not after what happened to Dad and especially after Mom was admitted for the kidney infection."

Joey looked at us all as if he was a proud father; he even said he was proud of us all.

Then he looked at me and said, "Fred, you barely touched your food. What's up?"

I looked at him with embarrassment and said, "I'm full. I can't eat anymore." Then, I thought for a minute about the servings or helpings I used to consume. I was sure when I loaded my plate this morning I was going to go back for seconds. I even remarked on that.

"Your body is adapting, Fred," Joey said. "You never needed to eat as much as you have all these years. Your body has been storing away as much extra fuel as it could in the form of fat, waiting for a long winter where there was no food available. Of course, then, as with the hibernating bear, your body would begin going into ketosis to burn all that stored fuel as you slept the winter way. This is the reason our country is the most obese nation in the industrialized world and the sickest. I'm happy that you are excited about this, Fred. Let's get you healthy and on your feet as fast as we can." When Joey perceived the awkward silence in the room, he realized his mistake. "I'm sorry, Fred. I wasn't thinking!"

I laughed out loud and said, "Don't worry at all, Joey. My doctor told me that since I was healing so fast, he thought he could fit me with a new and improved model within a couple of weeks. I'm looking forward to throwing away this crutch."

There was a perceivable sigh of relief in the room.

As we assembled in the den for class, Joey started talking.

"Today's subject will be about food," he said. "I'm sure Fred and Mother will remember a popular book published back in the 1940s by an osteopath and radio talk show host named Victor Lindlahr. The book was titled *You Are What You Eat*. As it turns out, this idea has been around for a few centuries. I did some research and found a paper dating back to 1826 by a French physician named Antheline Brillat-Savarin, considered the father of the Paleo and low-carb diet."

"He wrote: '*Dis-moi ce que tu manges, je te dirai ce que tu es,*' which translates to, 'Tell me what you eat, I'll tell you what you are.' This phrase is cited as the origin of the phrase and title of Victor's 1940 book, *You Are What You Eat*."

"What is interesting is that Victor Lindlahr started selling a weight loss and diet plan based on this premise even as early as the 1920s."

"Food has changed dramatically since the 1940s. The industrial age and the petrochemical age created a stockpile of deadly chemicals and toxins that poisoned our food supply as well as our water and air. The commercial farming industry depleted our soils of nutrients through the mass usage of pesticides and herbicides along with the continued commercial cultivation of the land, which we now understand destroys the 'microbiome' of molds, yeasts, bacteria, etc., that live in the soil and help the roots of the plants convert nutrients from the soil into absorbable substances to feed the plants."

"As a result, the food industry was forced to 'fortify' the food stuff they sell us. The joke is they used this as a promotional selling point, such as in the old commercial, 'Wonder Bread helps build strong bodies in twelve ways,' or, 'Wheaties, the breakfast of champions.' The truth is that they had to fortify the dead, nutrient-depleted food to prevent conditions like scurvy. The FDA allowed over

1,300, and today, even more additives, preservatives, and stabilizers to be added to our processed foods."

"Fast forward to today. So many people tell me, 'Oh, I eat very healthy. I only eat organic,' or, 'Oh, I drink tons of water and don't eat junk food, and I have for years.' Yet these same people are sick. They are part of the nation that has the most obese population in the industrialized world, which takes 50% of the world's drugs yet is only 4% of the world population."

"With all this in mind, I would like to suggest that it is no longer 'you are what you eat' but rather 'you are what you ate.' You see, the American population has bodies loaded up with toxins in the form of biochemicals, heavy metals, molds, hidden infections, and pathogens that just eating well today cannot get you healthy. We must pull the toxic load out of our bodies first, and this must be done systematically and carefully. What we have been exposed to through food, water, air, etc., over the years and down through the generations is killing us. It's a slow, painful, disease-ridden path to our demise. But something can be done about it."

Joey paused, looking at the three of us. The pause was deafening. Judy gave my hand a gentle squeeze as if knowing what I was thinking. I was anxious to get healthy now. I was ready to do whatever it took to claim my life back. I spoke up and told Joey and the group just that.

"Good," Joey replied, then shifted his attention to his mom and Alice. They both were in agreement. I felt a warm connection between Judy and myself; we would go on this journey together. "Okay," Joey said, "I appreciate the commitment from all of you. Let's continue."

## Glucose and Ketones

"Okay, for the last few weeks, you have collected and charted the reading of your glucose and ketones throughout the day. These numbers allow us to determine how well your body is burning these two types of fuel. I want to go over how each of the fuels burn."

"First, let's talk about glucose. Glucose is produced from carbohydrates and proteins." Joey must have seen the funny look on my face. "Yes, I didn't know that either. All proteins, either animal or plant-based, ultimately burn as sugar or glucose. And just to be clear, when I mention carbohydrates, I mean everything from French fries to broccoli! I don't think people realize this fact."

"*Glucose,* as it turns out, is a very inflammatory fuel. It burns dirty and has a lot of toxic byproducts that must be eliminated out of the cell and then out of the body. It kind of burns like wet pine in a fireplace – very smoky. If you shut the flue or allow smoke in the room, it would create a problem, just like if you had a hose stuck in the exhaust pipe of your car running into your car window. If this did not get corrected, you'd get sick and then eventually die."

"*Ketones,* on the other hand, are a clean-burning fuel. They burn like the blue flame on your gas stove – very clean. Ketones are not inflammatory. They come from the breakdown of fats and oils. We will talk about good fats and oils later, but for now, let's just consider these two fuels. One thing to know here is that your brains love to burn ketones! In fact, your brain is mainly made up of fats! Did anyone ever call you 'fat head?' Well, they weren't far from the truth."

That drew a chuckle, and it was nice that Joey was attempting to keep this light.

"Once we understand how these two fuels burn, we can make a conscious decision on which food to consume. We will have to figure out the correct ratio. But first and foremost, we must teach our bodies to burn ketones."

"So, how do I know how much fat I'm burning, and how can I speed it up?" I asked, anxious to get rid of all this stored fat."

"Great question, Fred. So, again, you are considered in ketosis when your readings are 0.5 and above. When you get to a five-day water fast, your ketones can go all the way up to even 5.0 or 6.0. Since you are not putting any carbs in your body during a fast (no meals or snacks), the only fuel source available is your stored fat! Well, there's also a bit of something called glycogen, which is stored sugar in your liver, but your body will be living predominantly off of your fat."

"Did you say five-day fast," I proclaimed. "You've got to be kidding!" Everyone laughed in the room, and I'm sure Judy and Alice were thinking the same thing. We all stared at Joey, waiting for his reply.

"Calm down, everyone. We will work up to it. Don't worry, you can do it. This is how you are going to get your life back!"

"And by the way, I just learned last week that there are ways to increase autophagy and stem cell production in as little as 24 to 48 hours. This is new stuff. I'm not completely educated on all of it yet. The cool thing about this field of regenerative medicine is that new discoveries and breakthroughs are being made almost daily. This is a very exciting aspect of it. I feel very fortunate to be getting this information firsthand and well before 99.9% of everybody else. This is why I tune into what Dr. Pompa presents to an elite group of practitioners weekly. I love staying up on this information."

"The predominate American diet is glucose-based," Joey continued. "You don't have to wonder why almost half of the population is diabetic or pre-diabetic. In fact, half of the people in this room are diabetic."

Well, there was no denying that, I thought, as Judy's eyes and mine met. But it went deeper than that. I could feel that we were looking all the way into our souls. There was a knowing moment when it seemed time stood still.

We were brought back to reality as Joey said, "If you two lovebirds are ready, we'll continue."

Wow, that was embarrassing. I could feel the heat running through my whole body, through Judy's hand, through her body, and back to mine again. We looked at each other and chuckled.

"Okay, so now," Joey began, "you will embrace the task of first understanding the damage done to the cells, cell membranes, organs, and the multitude of different systems in your body. You will also realize what you have been doing these past several weeks that is helping to heal your digestive system, which is necessary to allow you to repair your body."

"This is a list and sequence of the **5 Rs** discovered by Dr. Dan Pompa:

- **Removing** the Sources of Toxic Exposures
- **Repairing and Regenerating** the Cell Membrane (this includes repairing damage done to the gut or digestive system cell walls.)
- **Restoring** Cellular Energy
- **Reducing** Inflammation

- **Reestablishing** something called "**methylation**," proper detox pathway function, and healthy gene expression."

"This will help to turn on your good genes and turn off your bad genes, detox your body at a cellular level, and help to optimize your hormone function."

"But first," Joey announced, "lunch break!"

# CHAPTER 8

# Heal Thy Gut, Heal Thy Self

After we were all settled in, Joey brought up the topic for the afternoon. He started by recapping our conversation earlier in the morning and said he was going to expound on the concept of **turning back the biological clock**.

"Okay," Joey started, "I am very proud of all three of you – yes, even you, Alice," he said, addressing his older sister. "It seems you are taking this all in and managing not to bully me too much." We all laughed. "Is this making sense?"

"Yes, Joey," Alice said. "I didn't realize that somewhere along the line, you got smart!" She smiled. I could see that her old attitudes were slowly starting to diffuse.

# Leaky Gut Syndrome

"Alright," Joey continued, "so I want to talk about something called **Leaky Gut Syndrome.** So, the lining of your intestines has been damaged over the years because of several factors: bad diet (e.g., sugars, white flours, food additives, preservatives, added hormones, drugs, antibiotics, antacids, alcohol), prolonged mental stress, and various other stressors or toxins we pick up in the environment or consume along with the food it is attached to. The inflammation caused by these and other toxins causes a widening of the intercellular junctions, allowing large undigested food particles, microbes, and other substances to enter our blood stream rather than remain inside the intestinal track where they belong."

"The biggest culprit responsible for causing this damage comes from a company called Monsanto and the widespread usage of its product called Round-Up, or glyphosate. This product has not only been sprayed liberally on our gardens, fields, and around our schools, parks and roadsides, but also directly on much of our food supply, especially the GMO grains grown in America. We now know that this poison is responsible for many deaths and diseases."

"Monsanto has distributed over 28 billion pounds of the poison around the world since its creation in 1974. This tonnage has, of course, been sprayed on our poor planet. Glyphosate, by the way, is a major cause of intestinal damage and even weakens the blood-brain barrier, allowing dangerous substances access to our delicate brain."

"When you have a minute, look up Dr. Stephanie Seneff of MIT and her testimony in front of a U.S. Senate subcommittee hearing if you want more information about glyphosate and its drastic effects regarding the decline of our health. Diseases such as Non-Hodgkin's Lymphoma and many other conditions have been linked to it."

"Finally, a court case was won, and Monsanto was caught in the lie. They knew all along that glyphosate caused cancer, and they covered it up."

"It's not just glyphosate. So many toxins and chemicals add to the problem, and now it is thought up to 95% of Americans have some degree of leaky gut or intestinal permeability."

"Conditions that suggest someone might have leaky gut are vast: anything from colitis to chronic fatigue syndrome, fibromyalgia, anxiety, and depression."

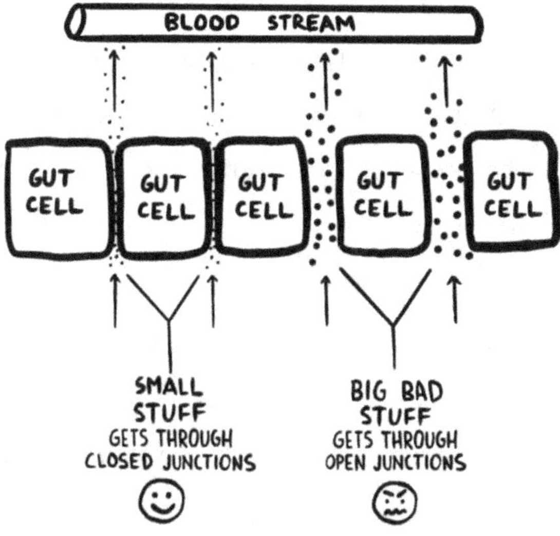


*Picture 16: Leaky gut syndrome*

"So, what do we do about it?"

"Heal the gut! The anti-inflammatory diet we embarked on will go a long way to repair the damage done to your gut. Not only will it tighten up the junctions between the cells, but it will also allow your body to begin to heal, tightening the junctions between your intestinal cells allowing only the right nutrients to pass into the bloodstream through the intestinal walls rather than the myriad of toxins and opportunistic bugs that have wreaked havoc on your health. Nearly 2,000 years ago, Hippocrates said, 'All disease begins in the gut.' Apparently, he was right!"

"So, as we continue our Cellular Healing Diet, which is heavy on fats and oils, the digestive system will become less inflamed and begin to heal."

"One other point I want to make here – and this is important – a tremendous amount of your body's energy is used to digest your food. So, if we follow the standard American diet or even the prescribed diabetic diet and eat constantly throughout the day, not only are we using up valuable energy, but we are also not allowing the digestive track time to rest so it can heal. Think about it: if you did pushups all day, every day, your arm muscle would become damaged and eventually cause irreparable damage."

"This coming week, you are going to give your digestive track a break. You proved to yourselves that you can stop eating for twenty-four hours, and it didn't kill you. Now, you are going to endeavor into a three-day bone broth fast."

"Don't worry. If, for some reason, you only make it a day or two, this is just the beginning of teaching your body not to depend so much on those predicable meals. Also, and very important, the bone broth is going to start healing your gut."

"If you are having trouble, I'm just a phone call away."

"During this bone-broth fast, your body will become less inflamed, and the gut wall can start to repair and regenerate. That is exactly what you are going to do this coming week. In fact, I believe that just fasting by itself, done correctly – which is what I am teaching you – will go a long way to healing your body. Why? Bone broth is not only loaded with several essential and non-essential amino acids such as glycine, glutamine, and proline, but it is also full of several minerals and vitamins needed to help nourish and heal your gut."

"Since you will be fasting, that energy that would be used to digest your meals can be used to fix things in your body, allowing it to heal at the cellular level."

"Guess what's for dinner?" Joey asked. "Bone broth." We all moaned at once.

Of course, Joey cooked his own bone broth for us. He explained all the different types of bones you could use. It was important, he said, to make sure the bones came from organically fed animals so we could minimize exposure to more toxins.

The bone broth was tasty, and I was impressed. He actually bottled up two quarts for each of us to take with us. He wanted us to continue tomorrow and up through Wednesday if possible.

He did say that we could have the keto coffee in the morning and fast until our noon meal.

Joey passed out a list of the different bone broths he recommended. He also pointed to the paragraph that allowed for different additives and spices to make the bone broth taste better.

There was also a paragraph on breaking the fast. He suggested fermented food, like sauerkraut, kimchi, and yogurt, as well as steamed vegetable salads.

As usual, the following week, I arrived Friday in time for dinner. We spent about thirty minutes going over our last week's endeavors. It was quite fun to hear everyone's struggles not to eat, but all three of us made it for the whole three days. I actually lost another eight pounds and was still not taking any pain meds. I was also sleeping well and noticed that my memory was improving. I could walk from one room to the other in my house and still remember why I did it for. This was important, especially when I was missing a foot!

That evening, Joey prepared a nice meal of a light chicken sausage spaghetti sauce. He served it on fresh squash, which he ran through a spaghetti-type grinder. Then he placed the raw yellow and green "spaghetti" in the bottom of a shallow bowl and covered it with the savory sauce he made. He even had some fresh parmesan cheese to grate on it.

I had to ask him how he made the sauce; it was delicious. He said he started with a yellow onion that he chopped and sautéed in coconut oil and some ghee, then added the fresh organic Italian sausage, carrots, and some chopped portobello mushrooms. As they were cooking, he chopped some bok choy and red bell pepper. He added a sixteen-ounce can of organic, whole, peeled tomatoes near the end, then seasoned to taste. I found out that he used chili powder in a lot of his cooking – not a lot, but he felt that it added an underlying flavor that helped carry this dish. He also added oregano and thyme to taste. One other ingredient was roasted fennel seeds. He would first roast them in a hot pan, then grind them with a mortar and pestle. All I can tell you is that it was amazing.

He didn't even have to precook the mock spaghetti – the heat of the sauce cooked it well enough.

# CHAPTER 9

# Our Toxic Environment and the Deadly Trio

I woke up feeling happy. I sat up in bed and wrote in the journal Joey provided. Following his instructions, I started writing my dreams and goals as though I was realizing them right then in present time, I composed my new life on the page in front of me. I wrote about how happy I was to meet Judy, Joey, and even Alice. I wrote about how Judy and I seemed to be falling for each other and how good it felt to be alive; I put into words how wonderful it is to visit with my family again and have my grandchildren sitting on my lap as I told them stories my grandparents had told I was creating my future life right there on that page, and I liked it.

When I got to the kitchen, I checked my numbers. Glucose was better, but still high, 135, but generally much improved. My ketones were 1.6. I was just sipping my coffee when Joey made his way into the kitchen. I bid him good morning and then mentioned my numbers. He was pleased and said that I was getting younger every day!

As soon as the group gathered and we all had our coffee in hand, Joey was eager to start today's class.

"Thus far, we have talked about how to reduce inflammation through diet. We discussed how to work to repair our gut, stop the continued damage to our intestines, and allow healing to begin."

## The Deadly Trio

"This next section is called **the deadly trio** and is a bit more involved as all three hang out together in the darker, danker spots of your body. In other words, they reside in places they should not be. I think it will be best to just go through them and then talk about what to do about the three, as they need to be addressed as a group."

"To begin, we need to address the damage done by the accumulation of toxins in our brain and body. There are three major factors first to understand, and then we will work to eliminate them from our bodies. It's not enough just to change our diet. We have to detox and pull these harmful substances from our body. But we must do it in a safe way. So many popular 'cleanses' on the market are either ineffective or even damaging to the body, just stirring up the pond, so to speak, but never really changing the bigger picture. It is important to have a thorough understanding of what we need to do. We can start by understanding what the deadly trio consists of and how to test for each. Only then can we intelligently move forward to remove as much as we can, again in a safe manner."

I looked at Judy and said something to the effect that it sounded like we were filled up with nitroglycerine and about to explode.

Hearing my remark, Joey commented, "Yes, it is true, Fred. This stuff is dangerous. Most of these toxins are stored in our fat cells. There, they are shielded away from the bloodstream and kept away from our cells and brain. So, when we detox and burn our stored fat, these toxins are released back into our bloodstream and can damage our cells, organs, and brain. Again, when we accumulate too many toxins inside our cells, bad genes can get turned on, causing genetic disease processes to begin. I can't emphasize this enough, we have got to 'Fix the Cell to Get Well.'

**Autoimmune**

"These toxins can cause conditions in which the body starts to mistake the body as the enemy and begins to attack itself. This is called an 'autoimmune response.' The body literally thinks it is the enemy. The National Institute for Health stated that there are over eighty chronic, often debilitating, and, in some cases, life-threatening illnesses that are considered autoimmune. They state that 23,500,000 Americans suffer from these, but in some circles, the number is considered to be much higher.

# Heavy Metals

"Heavy metals such as lead, mercury, aluminum, cesium, arsenic, and others are abundant in our current environment. The Industrial Revolution is responsible for the massive dumping of these toxic metals into the water we drink and bathe in, as well as our precious oceans, the air we breathe, and the land that grows our crops. We are exposed to many of them each day in staggering doses. If that isn't bad enough, Dr. Michael Skinner, an epidemiologist, says the lion's share (over four generations' worth) of heavy metals is actually passed down to us through our mothers' umbilical blood. In fact, the number one source of lead is our mother. – thanks, Mom. Lead is attracted to and stored in our bones."

## Lead

"Lead actually competes with calcium and has a stronger binding capacity than calcium, so it often displaces calcium in the body. Lead accumulates in your body where calcium is usually stored, such as in your bones. Lead has deleterious effects on the brain and nervous system. It also affects the heart and blood vessels adversely. The kidneys, digestive, and reproductive systems are also damaged by lead. A list of symptoms, such as depression, anxiety, and certain organ failure, can all be linked to the accumulation of lead in your system."

"The point here is that during the development of the fetus, all of the best parts of the mom are sacrificed for the development of a healthy baby. Since lead is stored in Mom's bones, when calcium is being called up for transfer, so is lead. The most obvious mental symptoms of lead poisoning are depression and anxiety. Not only do we get this lead dosage from Mom going four generations back, but we are also bombarded with it in today's toxic world."

## Mercury

"The second most abundant toxic metal – probably the most toxic of all – is mercury. We get this from so many sources, and for years, our exposure to this extremely toxic substance went unchecked. Silver fillings are 50% mercury, and for a long time, the dental industry stuck this within inches of our brains. We were told, and still are, that it is safe, but I recommend you start looking at the real facts. Mercury has been used for over 150 years in dental fillings, so this means that most of our mercury has been passed down through good old Mom. Again, thanks, Mom! Remember the 'Mad Hatter' in Alice in Wonderland? Well, back in the day, mercury was used to manufacture hats. The haberdashery workers would go crazy from the accumulation of mercury."

"The controversy goes on and on, but I'll tell you this: if you look up the top symptoms of mercury toxicity, you'll find symptoms such as anxiety, nervousness, irritability or mood swings, memory problems, depression, numbness, and even physical tremors. I think it is terrible that a majority of our children are receiving mind-altering medications for things like depression, anxiety, ADD, or ADHD without any investigation into the exposure and accumulation of these harmful substances in their bodies. I believe this oversight smacks of negligence."

"The deal with heavy metals in your body is that they love to accumulate in the worst of all places. Heavy metals love the brain, especially the endocrine system, and specifically the hypothalamus and pituitary glands. These heavy metals also hang out in major organs, such as the liver and kidneys. Even worse, they cross through the cell wall and enter the cell body and even the mitochondria."

"If we were only worried about the heavy metals, it would be one thing, but it's not. Heavy metals make the bed for other dangerous neuropathologic opportunists, changing the pH of our tissue and making a more welcoming environment for pathogens, such as molds, viruses, bacteria, and even parasites, to nest in and multiply."

"Well, remember that favorite villain, chronic inflammation? Well, that is the result of these unwelcome guests in our bodies' tissue. Now, a lot of us no longer possess a strong immune system, but even if we did, these bad guys are hard at work to create that dreaded phrase, 'age-related disease.' These pockets of toxic build-up incite localized inflammation to expound over and around an already inflamed area. The more inflamed our body becomes, the more likely this chronic inflammation will open the door to chronic disease.

## Our Toxic Environment

As we all sat and tried to enjoy our wonderful bone broth lunch, Joey reiterated how healing the broth was to our digestive system; it was filled with essential amino acids that actually worked to repair damage to the intestinal lining. Joey steered the conversation to other toxins we are exposed to. He said the lion's share of them can even come from our own home. As Joey went through the list of toxic products, I felt I would get sick to my stomach. He listed off so many products that I not only grew up with, but also still stored under the sink and in the medicine cabinet in my house. Raid, deodorants with aluminum, oven cleaners, disinfectants, laundry detergents – he said that even the fluoride in my toothpaste was toxic.

When Alice scoffed, Joey turned his attention to her and told her that all that makeup she was wearing was loaded with toxins. Again, she scoffed. Joey calmly explained that the FDA does not require cosmetic companies to disclose what they put in their products since they are topical and not applied inside the body. Since they went on, not in the body, the FDA did not require listing the possibly toxic substances. He told her to pull out any of her cosmetics and see for herself. Joey wanted to make a point. He said that even Diabetics know that you can put an insulin patch on your arm and have it absorbed into your body. So, why were cosmetics exempt? Alice defiantly stomped off toward her bedroom as we 'chewed' our bone broth lunch.

# Hormone Disrupters

"Some other things to be aware of are the industrial toxins used in furniture and clothing – not only formaldehyde but also the other 8,000 synthetic chemicals used in fashion manufacturing, most of which contain hormone disruptors and carcinogens. These facts are not included on any labels and are hidden from view in a sea of undisclosed pathogens."

## Xenoestrogens

"Polyester is a good example. It translates to 'many estrogens'. Synthetic estrogens are called xenoestrogens. Obviously, it is a hormone disrupter since xenoestrogens compete for the estrogen receptor site on our cell walls. Remember playing musical chairs as a kid? Unfortunately, when the music stops, these xenoestrogens take up too many receptor sites on the cell wall, delivering the wrong message. The long-term results can be devastating."

## Fluoride

"Another example could be fluoride in toothpaste. I'm sure you remember the Periodic Chart we studied in high school and that fluorine, chlorine, bromine, and iodine all exist in the same vertical column. Well, the primary mineral your thyroid gland needs is iodine. Just like the musical chairs example above, all four elements of that vertical column compete for the iodine receptors in the thyroid gland. If your body is saturated with chloride, bromide from pools and hot tubs, and fluoride from toothpaste, your poor thyroid gland doesn't have a chance."

"Today, over 30 million people in the US have been diagnosed with thyroid disease. How many don't even know why they feel so bad?"


## Aluminum

"The same thing can be said for aluminum in underarm deodorant and cooking pots. There are so many more examples, but the main point is that you begin to understand why our health got so bad."

## Forever Chemicals

"And now, as I have already mentioned, 'forever chemicals' called PFAS and PFOS, etc., have hit the scene. Substances like non-stick products for cooking, fabric protectors, fire retardants, stain removers, and more just won't go away and have been shown, even at low doses, to have deleterious effects on our health. And what's worse is, they are everywhere!"

"Now, I'll admit, it is a lot to stomach, but if you or someone you know are one of the unfortunates with failing health and no available answers, then maybe this is music to your ears.

"In order for me to help you truly reverse your biological clock, you will have not only to decide to minimize or eliminate these toxic substances from your world but also be willing to dig deep into your tissues at a cellular level to pull out the deadly trio."

About that time, Alice reappeared. She sat down, looking at us and then her brother, and said, "You are right, Joey. There is nothing on the bottle explaining what is in it. I had no idea."

"Most people don't, Alice," Joey replied. "That is one reason we are so sick; we have no idea what has been dumped into our environment. There have been upwards of 87,000 toxins dumped into our environment since the turn of the 1900s. What is worse is that few have ever tested for their toxic load. Also, many were created unknowingly as a byproduct of some other invention. So, today, the consumer must become aware and ask questions or suffer the consequences. It's clear the FDA, CDC, and even the NIH are not doing their jobs very well."

"There is hope, though," Joey said. "Pull out your cell-phones and go to the App Store."

Great, just what I needed. "I can barely turn the damn thing on," I retorted.

"No worries, Fred," Joey said. "Let me see it."

Before I knew it, Joey instructed the others and actually installed an app on my phone called "Think Dirty."

After recovering from the embarrassing name, I was able to pay attention to what he was saying.

"All you have to do," he was saying, "is put your camera phone over the bar code on the product you are interested in and – *boom* – up comes a rating on how toxic the product is or isn't. So, from this point forward – or until I release you back into the world – it is important that you use this while shopping. You can find out on the spot if buying that product is going to help you or kill you! Pretty cool, yes?"

Joey asked Alice to get the toothpaste in her mom's bathroom. When she returned with a tube of her favorite brand of toothpaste, one that promises whiter teeth and less cavities, Joey demonstrated the process of checking it for toxins. Voilà – it was loaded with them.

We all looked at the results. I must say, I was blown away to see that the CDC and FDA would allow us to be exposed to all these chemicals and other toxins.

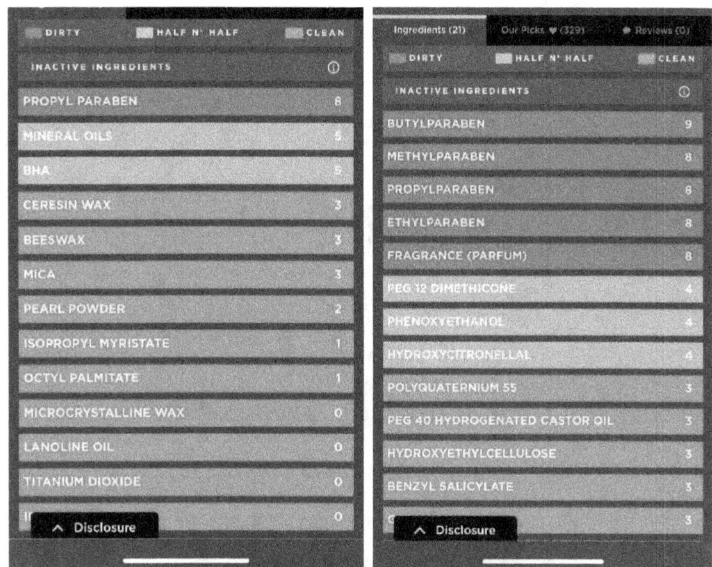

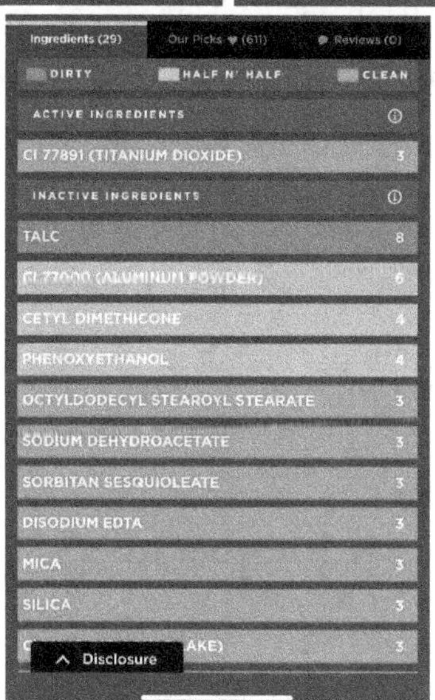

*Picture 17a: Toothpaste;*

*Picture 17b: Hair product; Picture 17c: Lipstick*

# Of Molds and Hidden Infections

"Molds and hidden infections are two more of the most important issues to review; if they're not known about, searched for, and handled, they could leave you suffering needlessly into the future. Mold is everywhere, and when someone is exposed to it, they can have a boatload of trouble getting rid of it. When mold takes hold, it won't let go. The other issue: hidden infections can be so insidious that they can go undetected for years, wreaking havoc on the systems, organs, and cells of your body, causing a myriad of symptoms from severe debilitation to just general malaise. The point is, who do you go to get these things figured out? I almost said 'to get diagnosed,' but where has the diagnosis ever gotten us? Usually, a medication to cover up the symptom. You deserve more."

"These three issues – heavy metals, molds, and hidden infections – can culminate in chronic inflammation locally or systemically and are most likely at the core of the plethora of chronic diseases in our country, if not the world. Some empirical evidence is the fact that we have more available drugs than any other industrialized nation in the world but are the sickest of all nations in the industrialized world."

"It is important," Joey continued, "to understand that the more you are exposed to these environmental chemicals, heavy metals, molds, and hidden infections, the more they are absorbed into your tissues, cells, and even your brain. Understand that it is not just these chemicals and metals you need to be concerned with; their presence in your body exposes you to a much greater threat. You see, they not only set up your body's biological environment to welcome in the deadly molds that surround us but also create a breeding ground for bacteria, viruses, and other microbes to take hold and establish infections. These infections can lay concealed deep in your mouth, organs, tissues, nervous system, almost anywhere. They leak mycotoxins, their excrement, into your circulatory and lymphatic systems. Eventually, they permeate your organs, brain, and tissues down to a cellular level and contribute to the expression of 'bad genes,' culminating in the failing health of our nation."

## Mold

"Mold even has its own passage in the Bible. In Leviticus 14, God told Moses to inspect the house for mildew. If he found it, he would get a priest to come and inspect it. If the priest suspected bad mold, he would have Moses get it removed and disposed of. God was clear that after seven days, the priest was to reinspect for mildew. If he found the mildew again, the house would be torn down, the timbers and any furniture or clothing in the house would be burned, and any stones would be buried deep and away from town. Mold is tenacious and takes a stronghold in and on the body."

"Mold is dangerous because it hides out in dark corners of your body and excretes mycotoxins. These are like the excrement of these little life colonies. They are toxic and insidious. They are the source of so many illusive symptoms and chronic diseases yet go untested and undiscovered by many practitioners. I'm not sure why they are so overlooked; they just are."

"For now," Joey said, "the best thing to do is inspect your homes for hidden molds. We can even have your house tested to see if there are spores in your home, what kind they are, how toxic they are, and at what level they are. We can test you as well. There are many tests out there – some are kind of expensive, so let's not jump to the gun yet. We can figure out what testing, if any, to do as we progress."

"Again," Joey reiterated, "not everybody on the planet needs to do all these things, but if your health is failing or you are just sick and tired of being sick and tired and have found no answers, maybe this is an avenue for you to explore."

*(See appendix for recommended tests.)*

Joey continued. "Hidden infections are an amazingly overlooked condition across the board when one suffers from a chronic disease. The source of these hidden infections could fool you. A friend of mine named Janet was suffering from some chronic condition for quite a while; she was not in good shape. She worked on everything from dieting to heavy metal detoxification, intermittent fasting, and the ketogenic diet. She even had a kidney infection that would not respond to nutrition or antibiotics, so she had to have surgical intervention. Finally, her chiropractor introduced her to a biological dentist in town, recommending she get what is called a cone-beam or three-dimensional x-ray of her mouth, which is essentially a CAT scan of her jaw. As was suspected, she had a terrible hidden infection deep in her jawbone at the spot of extraction of one of her wisdom teeth, which was pulled many years earlier. Cavitations are more common than one might think and can develop in root canals or even, as in her case, at the site of old tooth extractions."

"There is a ligament that holds the tooth in its socket called the periodontal ligament. Oftentimes, when there is an extraction, this ligament is neglected. As the gum heals over, this ligament dies in the wound area and then basically rots or necroses buried deep in the jawbone. This creates an unhealthy environment perfect for those opportunistic pathogens to make their beds, and they do. Recently, I saw the pathology reports of two patients; one was the woman I was just speaking of, and the other report was of a colleague of mine who was having unresolved health issues. Both had at least eight highly dangerous bacteria well above the 'safe' level that took up residence in these lesions."

"The 'cavitation' and its occupants start to create a manufacturing plant of 'mycotoxins,' which are slowly and clandestinely excreted into your body's lymph system. These toxins amplify any condition you have and even work to alter the genes in your cells, turning on bad things such as cancers, Alzheimer's disease, and Parkinson's disease, to name a few. When our genes get altered, a myriad of 'age-related diseases' can develop. Any of these inflammatory situations will increase pain symptoms due to the toxin's irritability on the body's tissue."

"I'm going to recommend that all three of you get a cone beam X-ray done, especially Mom and Fred. You both have diabetes at the very least, and I suspect you might have a cavitation as well. Let's rule that out. Oh, and by the way, the worst thing you could do is try to correct cavitation without first detoxing a huge amount of the toxins out of your body. It is imperative that you detox correctly and thoroughly before adding more toxins to your circulatory system. Because of the viruses, bacteria, molds, Lyme disease, and other pests that reside in your mouth, cavitation can be virulent. You must take precautions. Imagine finding a mouse nest in your garage. If you disturb it, the mice scurry away to the next best hiding place until they feel safe enough to emerge. This is exactly what these pathogens do once evicted from their comfortable home. And believe me, these things can make you sick. And if you are already in a bad way, this could push you over the edge."

(Below) Bacteria that was found in the cavitation ("hidden infection") of my friend's jaw. This was a failed root canal. Notice anything above 9 is pathological and dangerous.

<table>
<tr><th>Sample Collected</th><th>Sample Received</th><th>Sample Tested</th><th>Test Reported</th></tr>
<tr><td>08/03/2017</td><td>08/25/2017</td><td>09/28/2017</td><td>09/28/2017</td></tr>
</table>

**Sample Type: #17 Cavitation**

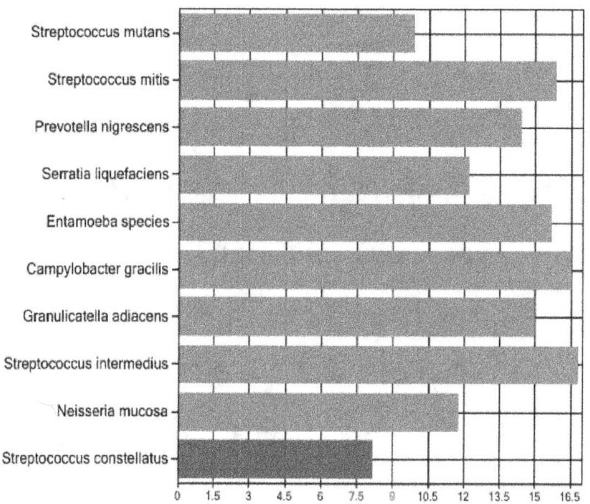


9 or greater indicates a serious risk

**Greater than 7.5 but less than 9 indicates a moderate risk**

Total Risk Factor, as reported on the chart above, is the sum of the Pathogen Risk Factor and Measured Risk Factor. Total Risk Factor equal to or greater than 9 is considered a serious risk. Total Risk Factor between 7.5 and 9 is considered of moderate risk.

Pathogen Risk Factor is the innate risk of the microbe based on the biology of the organism, disease causation, and microbial antibiotic resistance. It is reported on a scale of 1-10, with 10 being most serious and 1 most benign.

*Picture 18: Cavitation from Failed Root Canal*

With that, Joey announced it was time for lunch. When I asked somewhat hesitantly what was on the menu, he enthusiastically replied, "Why, beef bone broth. I'm sure you will love it!"

Judy looked at me and said, "Sounds appetizing." We all laughed.

"So, you see," Joey concluded, "if we are to regain our health, we must eliminate the deadly trio from our bodies and restore proper function once again. But worry not, this may seem too ominous an ordeal, but it's not, for we have our body's innate intelligence on our side. And remember - the greatest physician who ever lived lives right inside you. And also remember what B.J. Palmer said, 'The body heals from above down inside-out.'"

With that, we adjourned for the evening. I think we were all exhausted. I personally felt like I was fighting an overwhelming battle with an unseen and hitherto unknown foe. And yet, today, I had hope. Joey ignited in me a great desire – a desire to live and to love – and I knew at that moment that it was possible. I knew, for sure, I could do it. I could get my life back, and it was possible for me to turn back my biological clock!

That evening, we dined on roast chicken, a vegetable-ridden salad, and a butter-laden sweet potato. It was a quiet meal. I think we all were exhausted, yet somehow, we all felt the comfort of each other's company.

# CHAPTER 10

# Hormones Optimization – The Ultimate Goal

I continued to sleep better than I had in years. I was beginning to understand that the cleaner my body became, the less toxic it was, the healthier I would become.

Joey reiterated that by eating non-inflammatory foods and the right proportions of fats, carbs, and protein, my body was more likely to function better. He reiterated that as the cell walls became healthier and more functional, hormone receptor sites were more available, allowing hormones to get to the cells and deliver their message so that the cells could do their job.

"Okay, class, let's go learn about hormones!" Joey said. Off we went, back to the living room for another day of learning.

# ENDOCRINE SYSTEM

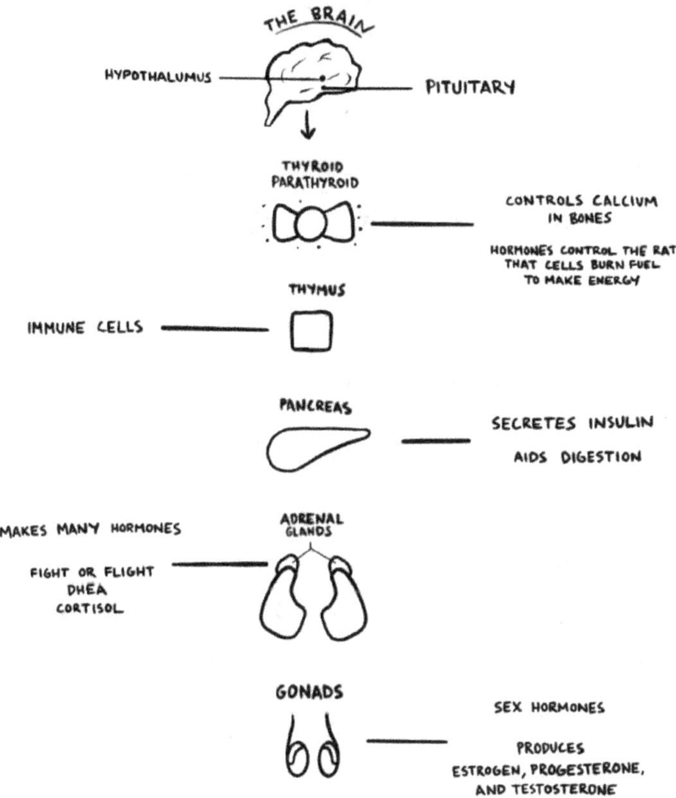


*Picture 19: Endocrine system*

Joey started to draw this diagram on the board to help us understand a bit about hormones and the endocrine system.

"As I have mentioned before, hormone optimization is the key," he began. "In fact, the main reason you all are feeling better is because we were able to reduce inflammation in your body simply by changing the foods you eat and how often you eat them. The change can happen that fast."

"By reducing the inflammatory foods, chemical toxins, and even the mental stress in your lives and bodies, your digestive or elimination system can do its job and clean up the environment."

"Do you remember the drawing of the cell I did the other day, or better yet, the video by Dr. Bruce Lipton I played? Well, that is exactly what we did and will continue to do - clean up your environment and detoxify your body."

"As your liver and kidneys and even your lungs and skin continue to dump toxins, and as you continue to put only the good stuff in, your body will become cleaner and healthier. Imagine a bucket of dirty water. Let's say you put a garden hose in and turned it on at a slow stream. Eventually, enough water would flow through the hose, into the bucket, and over the side so that the water in the bucket would become clean. This is how the detox works. By doing this through the different methods I will teach you, and based on your individual needs, we can help your body do what it does best - heal."

## How Full Is Your Cup?

"Imagine three glasses of water: one half-full, one full, and the other overflowing. Let's say the full one represents your body filled to the brim with toxins – a high toxic load. Your body is at the breaking point. One more drip of toxin, and you are over the top. Perhaps first, some symptoms, then a disease process begins: frank disease! These toxins create chronic inflammation, which creates chronic dis-ease. The toxins in the cell and the cell power plant (the mitochondria) get poisoned, and bad genes can be turned on in the cells, resulting in genetic disease. These diseases are not inevitable; genes must be 'expressed' or turned on."

"People in this scenario with at least one chronic disease diagnosed make up over 50% of our population."

"On the other hand, people with half-full cups (or empty) can handle environmental toxins and stressors much easier. Their body's detox systems are in much better shape, and they typically do not have a tremendous amount of chronic inflammation. And even if they do have some issues or get exposed to some stressors, like a virus, bacteria, or environmental toxin, the body can handle it. This is called survival. Our bodies have been doing a pretty good job of it over the years."

"Our bodies do have limitations, though. If you bury them too deep, throw them too high up in the atmosphere, get them too hot or cold, take away their oxygen, or hold them under water too long, they die. Even too much mental anguish, one of the three major stressors, can kill you."

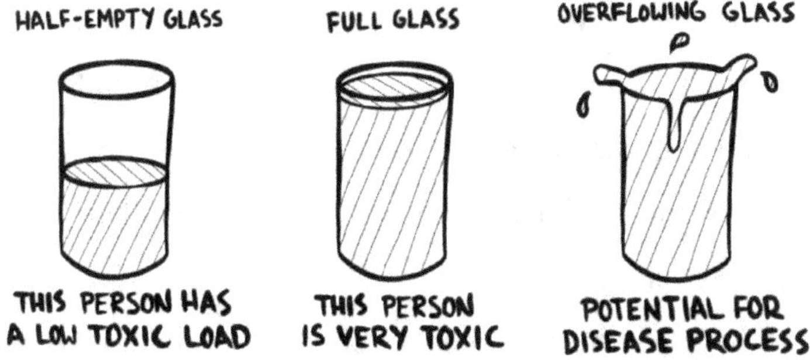



*Picture 20: What's your toxic load?*

"Whether you have good genes or bad genes, you are still better off getting your body healthy."

"As I mentioned previously, toxins can come down through four generations through mom's umbilical blood. The Environmental Working Group is an organization that tested the umbilical blood of babies who had not yet lived outside of the womb. They reportedly found something like 278 chemicals and toxins in that blood. Again, these kids weren't even born yet. Each generation not only gets their own lifetime exposure but also comes into this world with a boatload of their mother's, mother's, mother's toxins. Pretty crazy, no?"

"So, Fred, Mom, Alice - all three of you stated you are already feeling better in just a few weeks of changing your diets. We are eating less often and eating anti-inflammatory foods. We are also eating a lot of healthy fats and oils. In fact, I ensured that each of you was consuming at least six tablespoons of healthy oils a day.

"So, we cleaned up your internal environment and the areas around your cells. This allowed your cell receptor sites to free up so that your body's hormones are enough to act on the cells and create the desired result. Doesn't this make a lot more sense than ignoring the toxic build-up or, through a ton of medications aimed at fixing the symptoms, dumping synthetic hormones into the body to hopefully overpower the receptor sites so the hormones can act on the cell? I get tired, even thinking about how hard the body has to work to do this."

"Imagine if every time your car had something go wrong, you just jerry-rigged it. You know, if there is a leak in the window, you put duct tape; a leak in the radiator, you get some of that stuff that will plug the leak; your seats wear out, you put seat covers on them; your engine leaks oil, you just check your gas and fill the oil at the gas station; your car blows blue smoke, you drive the back roads; your windshield wipers are worn, you hope it doesn't rain. You get the point. This is how at least half of the people in this country are living their lives. It's terrible..."

"The truth is, nobody is telling them about this. The CDC, FDA, and NIH – all the powers that be – seem to have a vested interest in our country being sick."

"I'll tell you what I decided five years ago while standing in that stinky doctor's office with my dad and all those other sick people: 'If it's to be, it's up to me.' And I'll tell you what, it's up to you too!"

*Wow*, I thought, *what a morning*. I was beginning to get this. It all made so much sense. But I felt a bit pissed off. Here I am, sixty-three years old, minus a foot, overweight, toxic, prescribed six different medications, and this was the first time in all these years I even heard about this. Why don't they teach this in school, or why didn't my medical doctor insist I learn this before I opted to take drugs?

When I said as much to the group, they all expressed their protests and frustration as well after Judy's first husband and her kids' father succumbed to this very thing. At the same time, I realized that even this information may not be enough to persuade people to change. They will usually just go along in life thinking, "It won't happen to me."

Joey said, "You know, it's kind of like when there is an accident on the freeway. Everyone slows down to look; everyone is affected by the slowed traffic, and it could take hours to get through. But regardless, probably not one person passing by thinks about the fact that it could have been them in that accident. They typically don't pay attention until some get ill or get some dreaded disease."

He was right! I didn't! Too many Americans are walking around so toxic with hormone dysregulation and nutritional deficiencies that, amazingly, we are alive at all!

# CHAPTER 11

# Where Do We Go from Here?

I woke up early again, and my mind was running wild. Not only was I excited about the prospect of living again, but I was also happy about the possibility of creating my own life with Judy. After class last night, the two of us made our way to the little cement bench surrounded by primroses and cyclamen. There was a fantastic flower scent, and Judy said it was a blend of pittosporum, also known as 'mock orange' and night-blooming jasmine. It was enchanting. I must say, it had been years since I enjoyed a garden. My first wife Sara and I loved to garden and would spend weekends playing in the dirt. Somehow, being with Judy alone made me feel young again. I felt like Sara was looking down with approval.

Sara told me on her deathbed to find someone to be with, but by that time, I enjoyed alcohol too much and never felt very social. Thinking back now, I wondered how many people my age had just faded into the sunset, dreams never imagined and lonely days following them to a lonely grave.

Judy ignited a new fire in me, and I felt like I was living. It seemed funny that I had to fall so low to actually find freedom.

Judy and I talked until after midnight. Then, I told her how much I loved being with her, but I wanted to be the responsible party and get us to bed.

"We have class tomorrow, and I need my beauty sleep," I said.

She chuckled, and as we made our way back to the house, she put her arm through mine. It was a special moment; I don't think I'll ever forget it.

She stopped our forward progress by pulling back on my arm back. She turned, facing me. She looked up and told me she had not been this happy since she could remember. I felt weak in the knees but pulled myself together. I looked her first in the left eye, then the right, and then my eyes looked down to find her parted lips. We kissed, and time stood still.

The next morning, as I lay in bed coming to my senses, I focused on my new life; how lucky am I to have had this second chance. Second chance with both my life and love. Why isn't this information readily available? Why is it seemingly stifled and not taught to our unhealthy nation? I was beginning to feel a purpose stir deep inside me. I wanted to help. I wanted to make a difference. Thinking about the health of the citizens of the United States, being the sickest of all the industrialized nations and probably unindustrialized countries, I felt sad. Chronic disease was rampant and stealing happiness from the unsuspecting citizens who were just living their lives waiting for the other foot to drop. Oops, I had to laugh, for I only had one left.

But really, weren't there government agencies and organizations supposed to guide, look after, and protect the citizens regarding health and disease? What about the CDC, NIH, WHO, FDA? Joey had asked us yesterday if we knew what the acronym CDC stood for, 'Center for Disease Control,' we all said.

"You are partly right," he said, "It is actually the 'Centers for Disease Control and Prevention.' Well, I don't know about you", he continued, "but they don't seem to be preventing much of anything, except perhaps preventing the establishment of a better educational system for the populous on how to be and stay healthy. Also, why does the title have the word 'Control' rather than 'Eradication'?"

Apparently, there is also a Senate committee called the Senate Committee on Health, Education, Labor, and Pensions. What the hell are they doing to educate the people about health? Hum.

My bedroom was right off the kitchen. I could hear that someone was up, but there was no evidence of breakfast being prepared. I halfway was hoping to smell that beautiful smell of bacon as it sizzled away in the pan.

Reluctantly, I pulled myself up and made my way to the bathroom. As I splashed water on my face, I looked in the mirror and smiled. Even though I didn't smell bacon, I knew that within the next half hour, I would be sitting next to Judy, and that was exciting.

And so, it came to pass. Shortly, we were sitting side-by-side, hand-in-hand, ready for our new lesson on creating a new life. That is what it seemed to be, anyway.

When Joey appeared, he carried a box containing several smaller boxes.

"You've spent the last several weeks not only converting your body to burning ketones and glucose, but you have also unloaded a tremendous amount of toxins and made your body less inhabitable for the deplorables. They being the causes of toxicity, molds, heavy metals, and hidden infection, basically the source and cause of chronic inflammation, which we now understand is the primary cause of chronic disease."

"These –" Joey indicated to what was in his arms "– are some of the tests you should consider taking so that we can determine the best way to move forward on your individual health program."

## Telomeres – The Long and Short of It!

"We already sent in our 'telomere test' to find out how old our bodies perceived themselves to be. You will find that your chronological age and your biological age will differ. This is one reason why some people appear to age so much faster, and some still seem to be young even when they are up in years.

"The other major factor of this aging process is how the environment (stress) is affecting the body – all three types of stress: physical, chemical, and emotional/mental.

"These three stressors, once identified, can be altered, removed, or reduced with various techniques. As you reduce or remove them, the body – which is constantly regenerating itself anyway – can get ahead of the curve and actually make your body younger. We now know that your telomeres – the things that dictate longevity – can be lengthened through intermittent fasting and the ketogenic diet. When you add in all the other bio-hacks, diet variation, ancient healing strategies, and cellular detoxification, you can not only turn back your biological clock but also improve your cellular energy, overall health, and quality of life.

"Wouldn't it be cool if more people knew about this? I would love to help more people turn back their biological clock!

| Telomere | | |
| --- | --- | --- |
| Tests | Results | Units |
| Telomere Interpretation | 8.67 | Kb |
| Telomere Percentage | 91.00 | % |

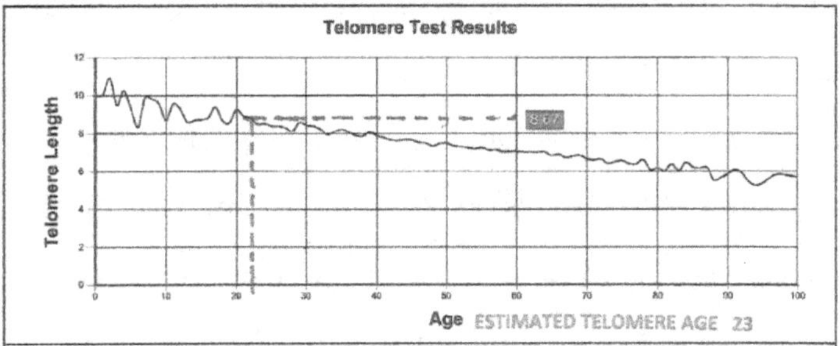

**Telomere Test Results**



Patient Average Telomere Length: 8.67Kb

Percentile relative to patient age and population: 91.00%

The Patient Telomere Score is a calculation of the patient telomere length derived from nucleated white blood cells obtained from whole blood. This result is graphed relative to the average telomere length of a sample population in the same age range. The higher the telomere score, the "younger" the cells.

A Patient Telomere Score that is above the black line (green box) is an above average Telomere score.

A Patient Telomere Score that is below the black line (red box) is a below average Telomere score.

*Picture 21*

*"Here is a telomere test result.*

*"... Attached is your recent SpectraCell (SC) telomere test (blood sample collected on 12/26/2019). As you know, telomere testing compares our chronological age to our average cellular age. Compared to our same-age peers, are we aging about the same, faster, or slower?"*

*"At the time of the blood sample, **you were chronologically sixty-64**. The SC test indicates **your cellular age (average) is twenty-three 23 (estimated)**. This 'telomere' or cellular age places you in the 91st percentile compared to your same-age*

*peers. Thus, your telomeres are longer than 90% of your peers. That is, your telomere age of twenty-three is the same as the average male in his early twenties! Based on cell replication, you are aging significantly slower than your age-related peers.*

*(These test results are actually mine, the author!)*

"At birth, we all have about the same length of telomeres (protective end caps on our chromosomes). As we age, our telomeres shorten at different rates. When a cell's life cycle ends, a new cell is produced, and through cell replacement, telomeres shorten. This is the process of aging. Once the telomeres are worn down, the life cycle is over. Telomere length is a prediction of your biological age and how long you may live."

## Heavy Metal Test

"Once we have given our detoxification system enough time to become strong enough, we will test for heavy metals. It's a urine test. Notice these mother-daughter heavy metal tests. Do you see how similar they are in lead and mercury? Even the cesium is identical. The mother was born in Pennsylvania and was there when the nuclear reactor at Three Mile Island melted down. The cesium is a by-product of that. You can see that the daughter's cesium level is remarkably similar. This is a perfect example of what the epidemiologist Dr. Michael Skinner was talking about: toxins passed down through the mother's umbilical blood. And remember, this goes back at least four generations, if not more.

This is why it is so crucial for young women who want to become pregnant to be tested for their toxic load before becoming pregnant. And depending on the results, undergo a detox program before getting pregnant. Did you know that the combined effects of lead and mercury are much greater than the sum of the parts? What I mean by that is that the combined accumulation of these two metals can be much more deleterious, dangerous, toxic, and either substance alone.

"We may decide to do a Gut Zoomer stool analysis. This test looks for the variety of microbiomes in our gut. Today, with all the stressors mentioned before – especially the antibiotics, medications, glyphosate, forever chemicals, street drugs, alcohol, and generally nutrient-depleted foods we consume – the broad spectrum of healthy bacteria has been depleted and replaced by a wide variety of disease-causing microbiomes. It can be important for us to determine the GI track's health regarding these bugs. This way, we can decide what to do to enhance the good guys while depleting the bad guys."

"Many people take a probiotic and have taken the same one for years. Unfortunately, this often creates a long chain of only a few varieties rather than a broad spectrum of different bacteria. An imbalance of the various bacteria or microbiomes in our gut can be responsible for the development of many disease processes. So, if you know anyone taking medication to mask or mitigate some symptoms or some named disease processes without assessing the spectrum of microbiome in your gut, they are more than likely just holding the symptoms down while the disease process advances. Eventually, you end up like one of the eighty million Americans diagnosed with multiple chronic diseases with no solution in sight except medication."

"And, of course, getting a complete blood panel, including all thyroid function and inflammatory markers, can be very helpful. This may be needed on a case-by-case basis."

"Other testing may also be needed, but our goal is not to spend thousands of dollars testing anyone to death, but to only do those tests necessary to know how to help the body do what it does best: heal."

"With all these test results, we will have a pretty good idea where your health is at and what it will take to get your life moving in the right direction."

# Provoked Heavy Metal Urine

# Mother

DCCTOR'S DATA Inc.

SEX: Female
AGE: 62

3555 Clares St
Capitola, CA 95010 U.S.A.

*Toxic Metals; Urine*

| TOXIC METALS | | RESULT<br>µg/g creat | REFERENCE<br>INTERVAL | | WITHIN<br>REFERENCE | OUTSIDE REFERENCE |
|---|---|---|---|---|---|---|
| Aluminum | (Al) | 7.3 | < | 35 | | |
| Antimony | (Sb) | < dl | < | 0.2 | | |
| Arsenic | (As) | 18 | < | 80 | | |
| Barium | (Ba) | 2.3 | < | 7 | | |
| Beryllium | (Be) | < dl | < | 1 | | |
| Bismuth | (Bi) | < dl | < | 4 | | |
| Cadmium | (Cd) | 0.5 | < | 1 | | |
| Cesium | (Cs) | 10 | < | 10 | | |
| Gadolinium | (Gd) | < dl | < | 0.8 | | |
| Lead | (Pb) | 5.4 | < | 2 | | |
| Mercury | (Hg) | 4.2 | < | 4 | | |
| Nickel | (Ni) | 3.6 | < | 10 | | |
| Palladium | (Pd) | < dl | < | 0.3 | | |
| Platinum | (Pt) | < dl | < | 0.1 | | |
| Tellurium | (Te) | < dl | < | 0.5 | | |
| Thallium | (Tl) | 0.2 | < | 0.5 | | |
| Thorium | (Th) | < dl | < | 0.03 | | |
| Tin | (Sn) | 0.4 | < | 5 | | |
| Tungsten | (W) | < dl | < | 0.4 | | |
| Uranium | (U) | < dl | < | 0.04 | | |

*Picture 22: Heavy metal test (sixty-two-year-old woman, mom)*

SEX: Female
AGE: 25

3555 Clares St
Capitola, CA 95010 U.S.A.

*Toxic Metals; Urine*

| TOXIC METALS | | RESULT µg/g creat | REFERENCE INTERVAL | | WITHIN REFERENCE | OUTSIDE REFE |
|---|---|---|---|---|---|---|
| Aluminum | (Al) | 2.7 | < | 35 | ▬ | |
| Antimony | (Sb) | < dl | < | 0.2 | | |
| Arsenic | (As) | 16 | < | 80 | ▬ | |
| Barium | (Ba) | 4.8 | < | 7 | ▬▬▬ | |
| Beryllium | (Be) | < dl | < | 1 | | |
| Bismuth | (Bi) | 0.2 | < | 4 | ▪ | |
| Cadmium | (Cd) | 0.3 | < | 1 | ▬▬ | |
| Cesium | (Cs) | 8.6 | < | 10 | ▬▬▬ | |
| Gadolinium | (Gd) | < dl | < | 0.8 | | |
| Lead | (Pb) | 5.1 | < | 2 | ▬▬▬▬ | |
| Mercury | (Hg) | 3.1 | < | 4 | ▬▬▬ | |
| Nickel | (Ni) | 4.2 | < | 10 | ▬▬ | |
| Palladium | (Pd) | < dl | < | 0.3 | | |
| Platinum | (Pt) | < dl | < | 0.1 | | |
| Tellurium | (Te) | < dl | < | 0.5 | | |
| Thallium | (Tl) | 0.3 | < | 0.5 | ▬▬▬ | |
| Thorium | (Th) | < dl | < | 0.03 | | |
| Tin | (Sn) | 0.2 | < | 5 | ▪ | |
| Tungsten | (W) | < dl | < | 0.4 | | |

*Picture 23: Heavy metal test (twenty-three-year-old woman, daughter)*

# Core Cellular Detoxication

*Note from the author*

*At this writing, I wanted to take a moment to thank you for getting this far. What we will be going through next is the New Dr. Pompa Program. This is the critical point we have been waiting for: getting your body healthy enough to even consider an actual cellular detox program that addresses the 'Up-Stream' cause of your health issues.*

*For the past 6 years, I have had the privilege to be in Dr. Pompa's 'Inner Circle.' Through this time, our group of 'Platinum Practitioners' have worked and studied closely together, participating in the evolution of this cellular detox program.*

*During our weekly Zoom meetings, where we brainstormed complex cases, broke down the newest research for clinical protocols, and then, if they seem effective, implemented clinical trials among ourselves to see if they work. We've been included in closed-door meetings with some of the world's most outstanding researchers in the biology of the cell, natural, functional, and regenerative healing, experts, and opinion leaders whom Dr. Pompa constantly puts in front of us. We've been invited to tour bio-regenerative farms, which are lands with at least six feet of virgin topsoils untouched by human poisons, fertilizers, pesticides, or herbicides. We've traveled to innovative stem cell clinics in Mexico several times and experienced the unbelievable advancements in stem cell therapies firsthand.*

*Basically, with Dr. Pompa at the helm, with his personal quest to 'fix the cell to get well,' and now with the release of the newest Core Cellular Detox Program, which I will explain below. We are now in possession of the most powerful, thorough, and effective detox program on the planet. And the research isn't stopping; it just keeps getting better.*

*We live in very trying times, with so many uncertainties in this world. One thing we know is the healthier you are, the better you will fare when the going gets tough.*

*When asked why he keeps going and is relentlessly pursuing cellular function and detoxification, leaving no stone unturned regarding the riddles of longevity, Dr. Pompa earnestly replies,*

### *FOR SUCH A TIME AS THIS.*

*As my good friend Dr. Mindy Pelz described being part of Pompa's World,*

*"It's like constantly being hit in the face with a fire hose, so much information so fast and at such a scientific and clinical level."*

*I agree!*

*Before I continue with the story, I want to talk about the newest product line culminating from years of research and clinical trials. I'll start with the introduction of two distinct nutrient extraction techniques. In order to understand this better, let's look at the age-old and traditional way active ingredients have been pulled from the source material called a substrate. So, a substrate would be the scientific term for the herb, plant, or substance from which we extract the active ingredients.*

*Now, please don't lose me here; this is very important to your understanding of how to really get your health back.*

***Extraction*** *technique - Age-old extraction of active substances using water or solvents such as alcohol, etc. It has been effective, but only extracting a portion of some of the active ingrediencies we know were available from the* *substrate. This has left much of the active and desired ingredient in the substate unavailable. It would be like knowing that there was gold oar under an impermeable barrier. What good could it do you?*

*The second way to obtain the active ingredients is **fermentation**. It is done with various yeasts and sugars. This has been very successful, except there is a problem.*

*Most of these fermentation techniques create a 'histamine' byproduct or reaction during the process. Histamines are very inflammatory and are known to increase inflammation in our body. Histamine actually affects some major energy pathways in our body and can overload our bloodstream with this byproduct, damaging our blood vessels and heart, to say the least.*

*Dr. Pompa has worked with scientists to utilize a 'non-histamine' fermentation process, allowing the active ingredients to be pulled out of the substrate safely and without harming our body as we try to do it well. These 'non-histamine' producing techniques also effectively pull out additional active ingredients previously unobtainable by standard methods.*

*This next process is utilizing the amazing mushrooms on this planet. Growing specific mushrooms on specific substrates has harnessed the most potent and natural extraction process imaginable.*

*Here is an example of how it works. For instance, the Lion's Mane mushroom can downregulate or reduce inflammations in the brain and gut cells. So, by growing Lion's mane on active botanicals, such as turmeric, ginger, or licorice (the substrates), which also have similar bioactive effects, we can significantly enhance those effects in the targeted area.*

*The mushroom biodegrades the botanical substrate and brings the active ingredients into the mushroom. So when humans now consume the mushroom, those bioactive ingredients are absorbable by our body. Pretty cool, yes? All mushrooms, not just Lion's Mane, have the ability to target specific cells and organ functions in the body. Each of the products in the Cellular Solution line has been created with specific mushrooms and substrates to increase the effectiveness of the response we desire. More will be discussed further in the story.*

*These three methods have created superpowered supplements found nowhere else on the planet!*

*There are a couple of other things that make these products unparalleled today. Whenever possible, we use ingredients sourced directly from our bio-regenerative organic farms. There are less than 100 Regenerative Soil Projects in the World today. Plants from these farms result in more active and potent bioavailable nutrients for greater effectiveness, especially for someone who is sick and challenged. Glandulars, also sourced from our bio-regenerative ranch, are 100% Grass-fed. These glandulars target specific cells, organs, and glands effectively. We're proud to be one of the few involved in 90 Regenerative Soil Projects worldwide.*

*As you probably know, minerals are necessary for almost all bodily functions, from enzymes and hormones to neurotransmitters and detox pathways. The minerals in these products have also been bound to proteins by enzymes to make them super absorbable to our body, reducing the effects of the indigestible minerals often found in store-shelved supplements.*

*Oh, I should mention that all of these products undergo specific third-party testing for toxic contamination as well as potency. Each test is reviewed and either approved or rejected by Dr. Pompa. This way, we know we are getting the strongest and cleanest supplements on the market.*

*End of the commercial break. And to quote my favorite Loony Tunes line:*

**"On with the show, this is it!"**

# The Plan

"So, here is our plan," Joey began, "Again, over the past several weeks, we have made major changes in each of your health statuses. Now, we want to determine the next steps for each of you so we can detoxify your body safely and effectively to optimize your health."

"We will continue the dietary protocol we have been using as we add in the Core Cellular Detox Program."

*Fix the Cell to Get Well*

*Dr. Pompa Cellular Solution Program*

"We will now embark on the new and improved Core Cellular Healing Program. This is a three-phase detox program that Dr. Dan Pompa put together. The three phases consist of:

1. the prep or preparation phase
2. the body phase

and finally,

3. the brain phase."

"I can't wait to see the results you all achieve! May you never be the same!"


## Cellular Solutions

"As all three of you are still adapting to the cellular healing diet, more specifically a gut healing lifestyle, I think we are good to begin The Pompa Program. These three phases of the program are designed to help all the organs, systems, and cells in your body begin to heal. I must say you are all fortunate to be starting this now with the new Cellular Solutions products."

"Just to get a better picture of what we are trying to do, let's review Dr. Pompa's Five R's."

The Five Rs:

- **Removing** the Sources of Toxic Exposures
- **Repairing and Regenerating** the Cell Membrane – including the mitochondria cell wall.
(Also repairing the damage done to the gut or digestive system's cell walls)
- **Restoring** Cellular Energy – Burning the two fuels more efficiently.
- **Reducing** Inflammation – throughout the body, but specifically at the cellular level.
- **Reestablishing** something called methylation, proper detox pathway function, and healthy gene expression to:
  - Turn on good genes
  - Turn off bad genes
  - Detoxify the cells
  - Reestablish hormone optimization

## Prep Phase

"The idea of the Prep Phase is to clean up our diet, which we have already begun, as we also lessen the burden on what has been called 'the downstream detox pathways.' These pathways include and involve organs like your liver, kidney, large intestine, bladder, and lymphatic drainage system, all of which are a part of your elimination system. By continuing to utilize intermittent fasting while following a ketogenic-based diet, we will assist you in enhancing your detox organs and pathways to regain proper function and allow for healing to occur."

"Based on your individual condition, you may be in the Prep Phase for a month or two. Mom, you and Fred should plan on two months. Alice, we'll see where you are in a month."

"If we move to *the Body Phase* too quickly, the body phase is where we start to pull toxins out of the tissues and organs. You could have adverse reactions to the detox, and we want to avoid that."

"The new Cellular Solutions line has simplified the amount of supplement needed, which will help you achieve this goal of opening downstream detox pathways."

## Body Phase

"In the *Body Phase,* we begin to add additional Cellular Solution 'chelators' to bind to and eliminate the toxins being released. This phase improves the health of the cell by supporting mitochondrial function, helping re-establish healthier cell walls, and, again, improving and strengthening detox pathways, all of which prepare us so that we can get to the magic of '*the brain phase. '*"

"During *the body phase,* we begin to pull toxins deeply seated in your tissues, cells, and organs. While supporting these various organs, systems, tissues, and cells of the body with specific blends of targeted vitamins, minerals, herbs, enzymes, amino acids, fatty acids, etc., all combined with specific mushroom compounds to improve absorbability and bioactivity. The body phase is designed to gently coax the toxic load out of hiding and into the bloodstream so that they can be eliminated out of your body."

"**Strong Binders** are the make-break point of successful detox. These are little understood, heard to find, and without them, trying to detox can create more harm than good."

"There are several different 'chelators' that bind to different types of toxins, be they heavy metals, chemicals, various pathogens, or even biological byproducts."

"Once the 'chelators' are bound to the toxins, it is vital that strong 'binders' are ingested at the right times and in the right dosage to ensure that these toxins are actually eliminated completely from the body. Apparently, some of the biggest dangers and shortcomings of almost all store-bought 'detox programs' are the facts that they are:

1. too short-lived to be effective

and

2. the 'binders', if used at all, are too week at binding the toxins and don't actually get the toxins out of the body. It's like trying to pick up a heavy metal object with a magnet that is not powerful enough to overcome the pull of the earth's gravity. The metal object will just fall off of the magnet and hit the ground.

All these quickie programs really succeed in doing is 'stirring up the pot,' maybe giving a temporary feeling of wellbeing and some temporary relief of malaise, but ulti-mately are ineffective in changing the overall health condition and quite honestly, since they do unleash toxins bound somewhere in the body, may cause more harm in the long run than good."

## Herx Reaction

"This body phase, and actually any phase for that matter, may cause some reactions called Herxheimer (Herx) reaction. This is when, as your body is healing, some hidden infections, yeast, viruses, parasites, molds, or bacteria hiding in your body detox too fast, causing symptoms such as rash, nausea, headaches, etc. Don't despair – we want these toxins out of your body. They are dangerous when laying hidden. These bad guys are excreting mycotoxins (their own waste) into your system, causing chronic inflammation and a myriad of complications regarding your health. That being said, please let me know if these 'herz reactions' do occur so we can mitigate them as soon as possible. This may be done by lowering a certain supplement dosage and slowing down the process or by ingesting

specific supplements targeting the problems causing the issue. These may target precisely mold, viruses, bacteria, or
some other pathogen or may include supplements to support or enhance the function of the organs or systems involved. This is the primary reason why people who try this
type of process fail or run into trouble."

"Besides the new Cellular Solution line, Dr Pompa has
created a toolbox of various supplements to target any of
the Herx Reactions when they arise. Remember, the way
out is the way through; the process works as long as you
let it go and work with someone fully trained in how to get
you to the finish line."

**Selfcare Dangers**

As you know, the body comprises 75 trillion cells, each
performing 60 million functions a minute, all controlled by
the brain and nervous system. Piecemealing various frag-
ments of detox programs or consuming bag-loads of supplements touted as today's next miracle pills can be dangerous and detrimental to your health. Selfcare based on
late-night internet searches often results in a collage of
non-related health protocols, frequently offsetting each

other, if not causing artificial or non-natural ingredient imbalances of ingredients. This can not only damage your organs and tissues, but actually can create adverse reactions in your body, resulting in chronic inflammation, which is exactly what we are trying to eliminate or reduce."

The major problem here is that people are desperately wanting and needing help. They have given up on Western medicine and are searching for hope and help out there. If Western medicine hasn't figured it out after spending 4.3 trillion dollars a year on health care in the US. Regardless of their motivation, what chance does an individual have spending their spare time searching the net or taking advice from a self-proclaimed alternative health expert to crack the riddle of the fountain of youth, turning back their biological clock, or reversing some chronic, autoimmune or life-threatening disease? It's a recipe for disaster. Get the help of a real expert, someone who understands how to 'fix the cell so you can get well.' Your life may depend on it!"

"One last point: when people try these helter-skelter remedies which at best may mitigate symptoms for a while but never get to the upstream cause, they eventually give up and either fall back into the medical model or give up hope altogether."

## Body Phase Continued

"During the body phase, we will be modifying your intermittent fasting and ketogenic diet programs as we have discovered that fasting during a detoxing phase can cause unnecessary stresses on the body. We want to avoid that. This will be based on your individual needs as your body releases the toxins. Each of you is different with varying pathogenic loads stemming from all the factors we have discussed regarding you and your family's history, exposure, genetic predisposition, toxic load, the size of your bucket, how you accumulated them, etcetera, so close communication with your health coach, that would be me, will be important as we add the different detox products and protocols. The Body Phase will last between two and three months. For healthy people just wanting to improve their health, it might be a month.

"The purpose of the Body Phase," Joey was on a role, so none of us said a thing, "is to pull as many hidden pathogens out of your body, I like to say 'from the neck down' as possible. Specifically designed 'chelators' will be added to your programs to not only pull the heavy metals and other bad actors out of your tissues, but to bind them up tight enough to get them out of the body successfully. We want to reduce the toxic load as low as possible so that when we move on to the brain phase, we can safely unleash the brain's toxic burden, feeling confident that it has someplace to go, that being, out of the body."

## Concentration Gradient

"The Body Phase is designed to create what's called a 'concentration gradient.' Since we have reduced the concentration of the toxins in the body itself, there is room for the saturated brain to dump or unload it's toxic load down into the body and then make its way to the well-functioning 'downstream detox pathways, a.k.a. the liver, colon, kidneys, bladder and lymphatics for final elimination out of the body."

## Brain Phase – Let The Magic Begin

"Our brains are primarily made of fat and toxins; all their friends and rabble-rousers love fat. As we start purging these substances from the brain, one of the first things people usually comment on is the re-establishment of their short-term memory. The brain fog begins to diminish, and your short-term memory returns. Imagine walking to the far end of the house and actually remembering why you took on such an undertaking, even remembering where your keys are, or suddenly having that scholarly vocabulary you once had."

"This is a big deal and may seem significant in itself, but remember, it wasn't getting better on its own and, in fact, was progressing, along with all of your other off-kilter brain functions. Again, by restoring a healthy brain, the 'bad genes' inside the nucleus of these cells can 'Turn down or turn-off'. This means, for instance, that any number of the 70 Alzheimer-related genes and other detrimental 'bad genes' found in the brain can go or remain dormant. Remember, just because we have those genes, we all do, does not mean you will develop that condition. If it did, we would not make it out of the womb."

"As we detox the brain, we also detox the hypothalamus and pituitary glands, thus reestablishing proper hormone function. Now, with the 'lower 48' (the body and all the cells and organs below the brain) cleaned up, the neurotransmitters and hormones coming from the hypothalamus and pituitary glands can act on the other endocrine or hormone-releasing glands in the body, allowing them to, in turn, release their hormones into the blood stream to act on the cells and signal the correct and optimal functions of the cells and organs they are communicating with."

"It is imperative that the brain phase is done at the correct time and done properly. These toxins have not only accumulated over a lifetime, but as you know, a large portion accompanied you from your mom's womb, four generations worth. So, as we release these embedded toxins (heavy metals, molds, biochemicals, etc.) from the brain, we must do it gradually. We can't just rush it. So we find it is necessary to rotate the brain phase with the body phase repeatedly, usually on a monthly basis, until we reestablish or, perhaps for the first time in our lifetime, reach our optimal health potential. Remember, our goal is hormone optimization, which is all directed by the brain, more specifically by the hypothalamus and pituitary glands, governed by the nervous system's interpretation of the environment. The number of rotations of each phase will vary for each individual. This will be determined for each of you as we go along."

"Dr. Pompa has repeated over the years, 'true detox takes years, not months.' But what is it worth for you to get your life back?"

Joey must have seen the forlorn look on my face, so looking directly at me, he said:

"Fred, you may or may not need more rotations between the body and brain phase than mom or Alice. Everything we have talked about, toxic load, the types of toxins or heavy metals, chemical exposure, length over exposure, genetics and the development of chronic and autoimmune disease, mental stressors, your microbiome, and digestive function, all of these factors come into play. Remember a few weeks ago when I taught you about Dr. Pompa's 'three-legged stool'? We are working this back and forth, improving each leg as we go until your body is unburdened enough and can take back the helm and do what it does best: heal."

"Remember, the greatest physician who ever lived lives right inside you. That is your innate intelligence. We must never forget that."

"Everyone okay with that?"

We all shook our heads 'yes' or muttered some semblance interpreted as so.

I was really beginning to understand what has happened to the health of our country. How insidiously these factors have destroyed our health. All the powers that be, government organizations from the CDC, FDA, and NIH to the special Senate Subcommittees have put corporate profit and their own personal gain over the safe shepherding of those they vowed to protect, those who put them into office. These actions or perhaps inactions by those bureaucracies seem treasonous to me.

I was reminded of the cynical Greek philosopher Diogenes of Sinope, who lived around 323 BC and was said to have spent his life traveling the land 'looking for an honest man.' I wonder if he ever found one?

"The new Cellular Solution products really shine here," Joey's voice interrupted my revere, "for with the addition of the mushroom extracted bioactive nutrients they have allowed for as well as for the bioactive actions of the specific mushroom themselves, the impart on brain function, and restoration is lightyears ahead of the game."

"One of the components of 'Brain CLR,' or brain clear, is something called ALA or Alpha Lipoic Acid. It is traditionally made or synthesized in the mitochondria of every cell in your body and helps convert glucose into energy. One of the cool things about ALA and the brain phase is the fact that ALA crosses the protective blood-brain barrier BBB and helps repair damaged nerve tissue. It also seeks out the dangerous free radicals that damage your brain tissue through a process called oxidative stress. Not only does ALA absorb heavy metals in the bloodstream, but it also helps transport other chelating agents across the BBB so that they can suck up toxins in the brain. This is an example of just one of the key nutrients used in the brain phase to help restore proper brain function, which will go along way in turning back your biological clock."

"Another example I have already mentioned is the Lion's Mane mushroom. This mushroom, grown on things like turmeric, ginger, and licorice, enhances the brain detox process as well."

## Glyphosate

"It is important to revisit glyphosate for a minute, you know, Round-Up, which is the poison from Monsanto I mentioned earlier. Glyphosate also has the ability to cross the BBB and, in fact, weakens and damages the BBB itself. The result is a widening or opening up of the protective channels or nullifying the locked barriers of the BBB, allowing many harmful substances to enter the brain. By opening up the BBB, glyphosate allows these bad substances to penetrate the brain and do even more damage. The brain phase is designed, in part, to help remove this substance from the brain and repair the BBB."

"By the way, and again, detoxing your brain is not something you should do willy-nilly, thinking you can do it yourself. You and your optimum survival are very important; you are worth spending money on; get help from someone trained in "fixing the cell to get well'. This is the most advanced, researched, and effective detox program on the planet. Dr. Pompa has nailed down the upstream cause of ill-health. Toxins cause chronic inflammation, and chronic inflammation cause chronic disease. The key to optimum health is detoxification at the brain and at a cellular level. You can take that to the bank."

"Okay, sorry for the outburst," Joey expressed, but we all knew he meant what he said, "Where was I? Oh ya, Like I was saying, once we have a lower concentration of toxins in the body, it is safe to begin then the process of pulling them out of the brain. Since the concentration gradient is lower in the body now than in the brain, the toxins are free to flow 'downstream' so they can get eliminated from the body."

## Understanding the Evolution of The Pompa Program

"Let's talk a bit about the unique properties of the new Cellular Solutions products, Core Cellular Healing, a.k.a. Pompa Program," Joey said as he produced a few bottles that appeared to be supplements of some kind.

"You see, when I was first introduced to Dr Pompa and his detox program several years ago, the 3 Phases were unique and very effective. This program was primarily formulated by Dr. Pompa and a biochemist named Dr. Shayne Morris, grandson of Doc. A.S. Wheelwright, an early biochemical pioneer who traveled the world researching some of the oldest and most beneficial herbal practices, including Native American herbology as well as traditions of China, India, Tibet, Africa, Polynesia, Brazil, and Europe. Dr. Pompa and Dr. Shayne worked together, continuing the research and uncovering the hidden keys to True Cellular Detox. A key component to the effectiveness of these products was the incorporation of symbiotic botanicals, such as specific herbs combined with the specific active extracts, a practice discovered and developed by Doc Wheelwright in the early days. These True Cellular Detox products and the 3 phase program changed my health and, thus, my life dramatically. You didn't know me then, Fred, but mom and Alice can attest to how much healthier I am now as a product of the program."

## Core Cellular Detox incorporating Cellular Solutions formulas is born

"What is way cool now," Joey continued, "is the fact that through continued research, Dr Pompa has teamed up with researchers in the world of the mycelium or the mushroom. Medicinal mushrooms have been studied for decades. Pharmaceutical research companies have been using them for years to extract key ingredients from herbs and other substances and create powerful medicines for treating cancer and many other diseases."

"Some of the mushrooms you may have heard of are Lion's Mane, Reishi, Cordyceps, Turkey Tail, or the giant Maitake mushroom, which lives on forest floors of China, Japan, and Northern America and can grow to over 100 pounds."

## Mycelia and the Mushroom

"Without going into a deep dive," Joey continued, "let me at least explain how and why these latest Cellular Solution products utilize the incorporation of medicinal mushrooms."

"What has been discovered is that by growing certain herbs and other bio botanicals on specific mushrooms, these little hair-like particles called mycelia help digest the essential ingredients out of the herb and such and turn it into much more absorbable nutrients. In other words, the product is much more powerful, and not only that, but hitherto unavailable parts or components of the plant are now able to be utilized and absorbed by the body. The implications regarding the increased effectiveness of these Cellular Solution products are evidenced by the rapidly expanding Pompa Program being embraced by an ailing world."

"So what was already very effective in restoring health at a cellular level has just been elevated to the stratosphere. You guys are fortunate to be getting in at the right time. May you never be the same again."

"It is important to note that the hypothalamus and pituitary glands, located in the skull, are not protected by the BBB. This means they are heavily exposed to toxins and metals throughout our lifetimes. The toxic build-up in these glands acts as something called hormone disruptors, which can wreak havoc on the endocrine system. It is one major reason people are so sick. Not only are they suffering from cellular inflammation causing damage to the cell walls, which can inhibit cellular function, mitochondrial degradation, promote genetic mutation, and any consequences accompanying this, but the endocrine system is also affected from the top down. These toxins disrupt normal endocrine function, which can cause so many disease processes to occur."

"The heavy metal and toxic load in the hypothalamus and pituitary disrupt their signaling hormones, creating unhealthy if not devastating effects downstream. These can include any hormone-related issues, such as thyroid disfunction (whether hypo or hyperthyroidism), autoimmune thyroid disfunction, fibromyalgia, chronic fatigue, dysbiosis, colitis, or even death of the gland itself; sex hormone dysregulation (failure to regulate properly) causes infertility; lack of menses, dysmenorrhea, painful periods, and endometriosis in women; and prostate issue infertility and erectile issues with men."

"Other endocrine glands, such as the pancreas, can be affected, furthering insulin dependency and other Diabetic-related issues. This goes on and on. So, the point is, let's get you through the program so that the healing can occur and you can get your health back."

"The results for me have been amazing and I'm sure the same will be the case for you all. All of you already look better and happier and have lost weight, and at least two of you seem to be falling in love." *Boom.* Busted. We all laughed, and Judy squeezed my hand, reassuring me."

*(More about cellular detox and the Pompa Program can be found at www.McCollumWellness.com)*

## A Trip to the Chiropractor

"By the way, if you are wondering about breakfast or lunch today, forget it! We are doing a twenty-four-hour fast. This means that since our last meal was at 6:00 p.m., we can eat tonight at 6:00 p.m. To keep our minds occupied, I planned a field trip! We are all going for a drive."

As we willfully piled into Joey's 1962 Volkswagen van – which was a beautiful thing – he informed us that we were heading to his chiropractor's office. Joey took the liberty of setting us all up for appointments, in which we would get a complete consultation of our health history, an examination, and a complete set of spinal X-rays. At that point, we would be done for the day while the chiropractor evaluated what was up with our nervous system and made any recommendations.

Now, I'd never been to a chiropractor; in fact, neither did Alice or Judy. But at this point, we were all game. This whole experience has been a complete eye-opener, and why should we start doubting Joey now?

The office was located in an upscale shopping mall in Monterey. Dr. Duncan McCollum met us when we walked in, embracing Joey and welcoming us to his office. The office was beautiful, clean, and elegant. His staff member, Natalie, was friendly and gave us the paperwork, instructing us on what to pay attention to.

Once we finished the paperwork, we were escorted to a large room with a TV. Natalie explained that the short video would explain what we could expect for the day.

The video was informative and explained the difference between pain relief, types of chiropractic care, and corrective chiropractic care. This was interesting, and I was fascinated by how the brain and nervous system worked. There I was, almost sixty-four years old, without a clue on how the body's nervous system worked.

Once the doctor was finished with my consultation, I was amazed at how many injuries he helped me remember and how many times I was actually laid up for a few days in pain just to have it go away and never think about it again. In fact, he had a poster in his office that said, "The six most common words I hear in my office are 'I thought it would go away.'" I thought that was pretty funny because I had that thought so many times regarding my Diabetes, weight gain, and many other health issues throughout the years. So far, the only thing that had gone away was my right foot. I had to chuckle at that.

The examination was revealing. Every time the doctor touched a sore spot on my spine –I don't know how he found them nor how he even knew they were sore, he would say, "Hum, isn't that interesting? When somebody has pain on palpation here, it indicates a pinched nerve or 'Subluxation' at this level.' Then he would push a button on this gismo hanging on the wall, which had a picture of the human spine, the entire nervous system, and all the organs on it. Whichever button he pushed would light up the area he touched, indicating all the body parts affected by that particular nerve. This nerve goes here," he said, indicating a spot that I would have pain, in this case, my shoulder.

Then he said, "Oftentimes, when a patient has a problem or a pinched nerve here', indicating the spine in my lower neck, 'they could suffer from something like shoulder pain, restricted range of motion, hand pain, or numbness, carpal tunnel syndrome, also these organs are involved, thyroid, heart, and lungs.' Then he listed off three or four other things that, invariably, I suffered from and asked if I had any of those symptoms or conditions. I did mention the asthma and now emphysema. Then he asked, 'If you had pressure on the nerve that controls your lungs, do you think it could contribute to things like asthma, a weakened ability to recover from insult, injury allowing a disease process to ensue? I suddenly felt like he and Joey were in cahoots.

Man, this guy was good. By the time he went through my whole spine, I was amazed that I was even alive. There was so much correlation with my symptoms. In fact, even the chronic pain I just thought was normal that was in my mid-back correlated with the nerve that goes to my pancreas.

Next, Dr McCollum told me he was going to do a peripheral neuropathy evaluation. Then he pulled out a test kit, the content of which resembled the tools one might see in a Spy film, which were used to extract secret data from the prisoner. I mean, they were scary. Pinwheels, needles, tuning forks, frozen metal objects, hair dryers, etc! Now, what had Joey got me into?

Of course, I was down to only one leg, so I asked the Doc if the test would be half off. This got a laugh out of the group, lessening my anxiety about what he was about to do. In the end, it was not too unpleasant and seemed to reveal the loss of many of my small sensory nerve functions.

Dr. McCollum finished the examination on all of us. As we compared notes, we all agreed that it was the most thorough workup we had ever had.

Natalie scheduled us all to come back the next day to review our x-rays and get our verdict! I was looking forward to seeing my x-rays and what Dr. McCollum had to say.

Again, I had never been to a chiropractor, and the experience I had was nothing like I envisioned.

When we got back to the house, Joey announced that we could now eat our one meal of the day. He said that we completed a twenty-four-hour fast and asked that each of us comment on how we were feeling.

I realized how good I felt. First of all, I wasn't hungry all day, and when I checked, my ketones were at 3.5. Joey said that was amazing. Also, I felt more energetic than I had for years, and my mind seemed sharp. In fact, I was amazed at how good I felt. Even the dull itching that I felt in my missing foot subsided.

Judy and Alice both expressed similar wins, and we all celebrated with a beautiful salad covered with chopped flank steak, roasted pecans, blue cheese, and a few blueberries. It was amazing.

We all took a break that evening and watched *White Christmas* with Bing Crosby and Danny Kay. It was one of my favorite movies back in the day. I had not seen it in years, and it made me homesick to see my kids. Judy must have picked up on it, for she snuggled close to me and put her hand in mine. It was a pleasant evening.

The next day, we were all up early and seemingly excited to return to the chiropractor's office.

Natalie greeted us as we walked in. She was so friendly; I rarely experienced that in any doctor's office before. She escorted us back to the office and explained that we would watch another short video so that we could better understand what was going to happen that day.

Once that was over, Dr. McCollum came in and asked if we would like to review all the X-rays together. He explained that this would be an excellent way for us to better understand how the body works and breaks down. We all agreed it would be fine. He started with Judy, then Alice. By the time he got to me, I think all three of us were becoming experts in the spine and nervous system.

He showed us what a normal spine should look like and then what ours looked like. I was blown away. The bones of my spine in my lower back were almost touching. What he called the disc between the fifth lumbar vertebra and my tailbone or sacrum was so close to being fused that the hole the nerves came out of was next to nothing. He pushed a button on the wallchart again, showing me that the nerve exiting the spine at that level not only went to my lower back but also to my prostate. What really got me was that the nerve also went all the way down to my feet. He touched a button on a wall chart that lit up the whole pathway from my back to my toes.

When I asked him if that could have been what had caused me to have sciatic pain all those years, he asked me what I thought. I liked this about him; rather than just throwing out information, he consulted my understanding. This was refreshing and in line with what Joey was teaching us. It was time that we took control of our health. To do that, we had to develop an understanding of how our bodies worked.

By the time Dr. McCollum finished reviewing my X-rays, I was not only thoroughly impressed but also totally understood that it was the subluxations (pinched nerves) and the degree to which the bones improperly wore due to prolonged misalignment that caused the spinal degeneration or "osteoarthritis" I had in my spine. I also understood that these conditions developed over many years and that a minor or major injury to the spine that never healed correctly would cause the spine to wear at that level, much like a tire that hit a curb on your car. Slowly but surely, it would wear out faster than the rest. He mentioned that, like a cavity in a tooth, you might not notice it until it's bad enough that it hits the nerve; then you know, with no uncertain terms, that you have a tooth problem. He said that because there are only thirty-one spinal nerves exiting each side of the spine and that they go to the seventy-five trillion cells, sometimes the symptoms seem unrelated to the nerves and may show up as organic issues, such as heartburn, gastritis, asthma, bladder issues, etc. He demonstrated this pretty well the day before when, on examination, he touched a place on my spine and then pushed the button on the wallchart, lighting up the pathway that particular nerve traveled, indicating the possible related symptoms. It was amazingly accurate, and I wondered why my medical doctors were never so thorough.

He didn't stop there. Next, he reviewed the results of my peripheral neuropathy testing. Obviously, by the time I lost my right leg, the nerve and tissue had decayed to the breaking point. I was hoping the doctor would have good news regarding the prognosis of my left foot.

Thankfully, Dr. McCollum told me there was hope. Even though the sensory damage in the left foot indicated a 60% loss, he assured me that he could help restore a good portion of nerve function.

Here was the plan: First, he wanted to jump on any peripheral neuropathy. For this, he recommended several things. There was this thing called a Rebuilder; he called it a biofeedback machine. It consisted of a battery-powered device with a lead ending in two electrodes. The electrode would be placed in a bucket divided into two sections. These would be filled with water. I was to put my feet in the bucket and run the device for 30 minutes each day. He said that the rebuilder sent a signal from the toes to the brain 8 times a second, reestablishing the nerve pathways much like walking through a field of grass. The more you walked the same path, the more established the path became. By doing this, the nerves themselves would regrow. He said the scientific literature proved that the peripheral nerve had the ability to grow 1 millimeter a day if the right conditions were met.

Next, he introduced some LED redlight boots. He showed me two different lights: the infrared light, which we could not see with the human eye, and the ultraviolet light. These were designed to reestablish something called the "myelin sheath". This apparently is the protective coating surrounding the nerve itself, both protecting the nerve and the capillaries within the sheath, providing the oxygen and nutrients needed to grow and nurture the newly developing nerves.

This was not all, though. Next, he introduced me to the Softwave Therapy machine. Wow, this thing was amazing. This device from Germany is called a lithotripsy machine. Translated literally to mean Litho =stone, tripsy = to break. It was originally created to break up kidney stones without surgery. In this case of peripheral neuropathy, it helps in attracting our body's own stem cells to the area of application, allowing for something called "angio-neogenesis", or the new growth of tiny blood vessels called capillaries. Everything involved in the peripheral neuropathy protocol was designed to either regrow the nerves or regrow the myelin shcath, which h protects and nourishes the newly developed nerves.

It was all so fascinating, and I was amazed that this was the first I'd ever heard of it. What about all the millions of people out there suffering from peripheral neuropathy who were stuck in a broken system, slowly losing their freedom and more?

So began my journey through corrective chiropractic care, including the peripheral neuropathy program. I received my first adjustment that day, as well as my first Softwave therapy treatment. Surprisingly, it felt amazing, and I immediately felt more motion in my spine and seemed to feel a bit of activity in my one remaining foot. Having lost my right foot, I had to adapt to a whole new posture. I didn't even realize how much chronic pain and discomfort I was in until it actually wasn't there. Dr. McCollum laughed and said it was common for people to live in so much pain that it just became background noise, and the pain just became part of life.

That evening, as we were comparing notes, we all were amazed at how we felt. Alice commented that she experienced low-grade headaches for years but never thought twice about them – she just took Tylenol when that got too bad. She said that during the exam, Dr. McCollum touched her neck just below her right ear. She couldn't believe how sore it was. But when Dr. McCollum asked if she had headaches behind her right eye, she was amazed.

"How did you know?" she asked. Then, Alice explained the same thing we experienced. "Dr. McCollum said, "Oftentimes when you have pressure on a nerve right here, it can cause pain right here," pointing to the exact spot of my headache, and then pushing the button on the wall, which lit up the brain on the chart. 'She said something that I was thinking myself: 'It was almost like magic.'

Then, she said something cool. "When he adjusted that bone, it made a loud pop that scared me for a second. Then, I felt a huge surge of energy into my brain – and my whole body, really – but what was really amazing was that the constant chronic headache I had for years just went away. And you know what? It's still gone!"

And so, we were sold. It was apparent that if we succeeded in turning back our biological clock, chiropractic and a sound nervous system were definitely part of the equation.

We all started our journey to spinal health together and, for the next several weeks, visited Natalie and Dr. McCollum for corrective chiropractic care. We were all looking forward to our follow-up X-rays so that we could see just how good our body could get. Dr. McCollum reminded us, though, that at this point, it was mainly about function and 100% communication up and down the spinal nerves. He mentioned that the worn vertebra would not 'un-ware' but that he could dramatically slow down, if not stop, the continued damage already done.

He also mentioned that the nervous system was responsible for reading the environment and sending signals to the brain. The brain interprets the incoming info and sends information to the hypothalamus; the hypothalamus then sends information to the pituitary gland through nerve connections and chemical messengers, which then send out hormone messages to all the appropriate endocrine glands via hormones injected into the bloodstream. He reiterated what Joey was teaching us: toxic build-up in our brain, hypothalamus, pituitary gland, and any other cells or organs in our body was a recipe for disaster.

He commented that Joey was well-trained in the Cellular Healing lifestyle, as well as in the Core Cellular Detox programs and that we were in great hands. He encouraged us to stick with it. He said that with chiropractic freeing up the nerves, with the cellular healing lifestyle helping us burn our stored fat, and with the Core Cellular Detox program pulling all the harmful toxins out of our bodies, we were on the right track and would be living in entirely different bodies within a few months time.

This would have been hard for me to imagine a few months ago, but understanding as much as I do now, it seemed possible.

I commented to my group and got agreement. "Why is this the first time we ever heard of this? And better yet, how do we help others learn what we now know? I want to scream this from the rooftops or even the mountaintops." I looked at Joey and asked him, "Joey, what can we do to help?" And so it began…

Just when I thought we had learned enough, Dr. McCollum insisted that we attend his orientation class. It was on a Tuesday night; so after we enjoyed our OMD or one meal a day dinner, we attended his class.

The main topic was one that mothers across America would be happy about. It was all about proper posture. My mom was always hounding me to sit up straight so not to be a slouch – and I still had bumps on my head from her reminders – Dr. McCollum related posture to the proper function of the nerves. This made so much more sense now. He showed us how much pressure was put on the nerves of the upper spine if you slouched your upper back. He asked us all to look at the other attendees. There were about twenty of us in the room. He asked if we minded him using each of us for a teaching moment. Then, he proceeded to evaluate each of our postures, both sitting and standing. This was such an amazing teaching moment. By the end of the meeting, we all understood what proper posture looked like. We all had a good idea of what muscles we needed to use to achieve optimum posture ourselves.

Dr. McCollum gave us all a couple of homework assignments:

- For the next forty-eight hours, no matter where we went, observe the posture of people around us.
- Every time we saw one of us slouching or displaying poor posture, say, "Thank you for reminding me to have better posture."

I loved this idea! Rather than try to correct each other, we simply thanked them for reminding us. It was a good trick and stopped us from harassing each other.

Dr. McCollum also gave us a link to his website, www.mccollumwellness.com, where we could find different videos and pictures instructing us on posture and other health-related material.

# CHAPTER 12

# One Year Later

Judy had been on the road for a little over a week. We visited several National Parks along the way. As we drove along, I could not help but ponder this past year and all I had experienced.

My life had changed so dramatically by just changing the foods I ate and when I ate them. I did have high heavy metals, especially lead and mercury. We worked to lower them by utilizing the Core Cellular Detox Program and the Cellular Healing Lifestyle Diet.

I was so happy. Having lost 80 pounds, I was hovering about 190. I hadn't weighed this little since college. The prosthetic worked amazingly well; Judy said I barely limped anymore. There were a couple of different attachments for hiking or jogging.

I reflected back to waking up in that hospital bed so many months ago, diseased, alone, and minus a foot. Who would have known that only a bit over a year later, I would be so happy? I'm off all medications, have no signs of Diabetes, have no high blood pressure, and have cholesterol and blood sugar within range.

My microbiomes were now in good shape. The first Gut Zoomer test I did was terrible. I was loaded with bad microbiomes. But through the process of first fixing the gut (leaky gut) by eliminating foods, drugs, and other things that continuously toxified my digestive system and by taking certain supplements to help heal the cell walls and reduce inflammation, I was able to reverse much of the damage done by my past lifestyle.

My telomere test showed my biological age at seventy years old, six years older than my chronological age. This meant that my cells were wearing out faster than my actual age. This was still an improvement because, the first measurement I did, my telomeres were at seventy-seven. So, in a little over a year, I decreased my biological age by seven years, and I wasn't done yet!

This whole experience was a huge wake-up call, and I was using everything I learned and was still learning to reverse this trend. I was now driven by a huge purpose –

well, two purposes - one, my new desire to live, and two, my desire to enjoy my life. I did not realize how far down I had gone. For the longest time, I was barely operating in survival mode and barely aware I was alive.

The truth is, now that I look around, I'm amazed at how "asleep" people are. They just seem to be walking around in a trance, following the CDC and AMA guidelines and medicating their symptoms away until they go away. Unfortunately, the majority of the time, when their symptoms stop, it is accompanied by the stopping of their heart. It was sad to see, especially when you know a way out. I felt determined to get my story out for others to read and learn about. I just felt too good not to share it.

The other major purpose was, of course, Judy. We were so in love. I never could have conceived it possible at this point in my life. She was wonderful and truly cared about me. We had an amazing connection, spiritually. Funny, I would have never said something like "spiritually" before. But going through this process together – both nearly on our deathbeds - slowly pulling ourselves literally out of the muck and mire of drugs and toxins, healing our damaged bodies, then emerging hand in hand as a

strong, loving, and determined couple ready to save the
world.

# CHAPTER 13

# Reunited

As we pulled up to the house, Judy reached over and touched my leg. "It's going to be fine, Fred. I promise," she reassured me.

We had been talking about this moment many times throughout the year. Even though I was hesitant, Judy insisted we go.

I parked the car, placed my hands on the steering wheel, and took a big breath. "I hope you are right, Judy. I'm a bit scared," I said.

"Don't be. Everything will be fine." She reassured me.

As I looked at myself in the rearview mirror, I saw a younger man, happy and healthy – a vast contrast to a year ago. The program Joey put us through was successful and became a lifestyle for us. I would never go back to the way I used to be, eating and drinking with no regard, with no understanding of how to take care of my own body and my own health. I opened the passenger door for Judy, and as she emerged from the car, I was stunned at how radiant she looked. She, too, transformed. She was lovely; the lion share of her long silver blond hair flowing over her shoulders with the last bit rolled into a bun held in place by decorative chopstick; a beautiful Japanese-style dinner dress with cranes and bamboo plants decorating the material; and her soft, loving smile showing me that all would be well.

As we approached the front door, she put her arm in mine and gave me a nudge. "Have fun with it, Fred."

The door opened before I could knock, and standing there were my three kids, all together, ready to welcome me. Behind them were their husbands and wives; interspersed between legs and arms were my six grandkids.

"Hello, father," Sally, my oldest, said. "You must be Judy. We finally get to meet in person. Please come in."

My world exploded when I saw my three children standing there, surrounded by their lovely families. My heart melted. In their eyes, I could see all of life, and in that brief nanosecond, I felt my whole world meld with theirs. It was going to be okay. They were there to share their love. A vast wave of emotion swarmed over my body as I was embraced by my family one by one, tears rolling down my cheeks and my body becoming warm with love. As we hugged, I could feel the hearts of each of my children as we embraced – first Sally, then Mike, and finally Sara, who was my youngest and named after her mother.

"I've missed you, Daddy." The words slipped out of her lips, and I could feel our tears intermingle as they freely rolled down our cheeks. "She's lovely, Daddy. Mother would approve."

As I introduced Judy to my family, genuine love and appreciation poured out of all who were present. I was so grateful. Judy had contacted Sally behind my back and started a dialogue with her. I guess she was at it for months and finally convinced her to gather the family to meet. She had worked a miracle because they had all been ignoring my occasional call for years. I alienated them so badly.

There was a cacophony of hellos and welcomes.

We had a wonderful visit. I got to meet my youngest three grandkids for the first time and caught up with the other three and what their interests were.

Everyone seemed to love Judy - who wouldn't! - and she showed them some pictures of our wedding. We had married four months earlier. We had a small ceremony with Joey and Alice as the best man and the maid of honor. We held the ceremony in a beautiful state park called Point Lobos. It is located right on the coast south of Carmel and north of Big Sur. It was one of the happiest days of my life.

But now, there they were in front of me. Sally invited us in. Her house was warm and beautifully decorated, and there was a huge sign that read, "Welcome Newlyweds." It was truly the best day of my life.

*And they lived happily ever after!*

# Final Notes

It has been a pleasure having you enjoy this book. I hope you were able to utilize some of the principles in it and that you are healthier for it. I want to mention that Diet Variation is one of the keys to a healthy body. Staying on one diet too long is not healthy and can cause more problems than benefits. Please be sure to find out about diet variations. A good plan, once you have reached your 'fighting weight' and restored the lion's share of your health, is to eat with the seasons. This is a safe way to ensure you are assuming a healthy diet rotation.

Also, if you shop at farmer's markets, which is highly recommended, be sure to buy from different vendors. The varying soils of their individual farms have different microbiomes in the soil. As you know already, these microbiomes digest nutrients in the soil, and plants can consume them. The healthy microbiome in our gut converts the nutrients yet again so that our body can digest them.

Stay away from all GMO foods.

Eat organic.

Avoid chemical exposure in your house and on your body.

Consume plenty of vitamin G. G for gratitude.

Try to avoid 'forever chemicals'.

Don't drink tap water.

Continue the detox process to help you but not accumulate the toxic burden that got you in the mess in the first place.

Thank you!


Much Love,
Dr. Duncan McCollum, D.C.

# Appendix: Glossary of Terms

*1. What is fasting?* Fasting is an ancient practice used by almost every ancient culture in the world. There are several types of fasting. Today, it is used as a weight loss tool as well as a way of healing the body by reducing chronic inflammation and, thus, chronic disease. When done correctly, it can be quite effective. It is best to follow guidelines on how to fast, or if you are suffering from some chronic condition, do it under the supervision of a healthcare provider.

- **Intermittent fasting** is basically periods of no food consumption. It can also be called a fasting window. This is usually an eight-hour eating window and a sixteen-hour fasting window. This allows the digestive system to rest and repair.

- **Block fasts**. This may be a five-day water fast or a three-day bone broth fast. These timeframes may vary depending on the individual.

- **Fasting-mimicking diet**. This is a way of consuming certain foods each day in a way that tricks the body into going into ketosis.

The three above-mentioned fasts allow you to drink water.

- **Dry fast**. This is a fast where you consume nothing, not even water, for a day or longer.

There are other fasts, but these are the main ones.


*1. How does fasting work?* Fasting, done correctly, allows your body to start burning ketone fuel from fat or oils. With fasting, your body does not have a plethora of glucose-producing foods (protein and carbohydrates) and, therefore, converts to burning ketones. This is what we are looking to achieve in the Cellular Healing Diet. Ketones burn clean with few toxins. The brain loves burning ketones, and the anti-inflammatory quality of burning ketones allows the body to begin to heal.

*2. Glucose*, as it turns out, is an inflammatory fuel. It burns dirty and has a lot of toxic byproducts that must be eliminated out of the cell and then out of the body. It kind of burns like wet pine in a fireplace – very smoky. If you shut the flue or allow smoke in the room, it creates a problem, just like if you had a hose stuck in the exhaust pipe of your car running into your car window. If this did not get corrected, you'd get sick and eventually die.

*3. Ketones* are a clean-burning fuel. They burn like the blue flame on your gas stove – very clean. Ketones are not inflammatory. They come from fats and oils.

*4. What is ketosis?* It is a state where your body is burning ketones for fuel. To monitor the degree of ketosis, you use a keto meter. Anywhere between 0.5 to 6.0 represents ketosis. You don't reach the higher number without a prolonged fast of three to five days. This is a healing moment.

*How does it work?* Every cell in our body – except maybe red blood cells – has the ability to burn ketones. When you are in ketosis, you gradually and safely reduce the carbs and protein to the point that the "old ketone burners," packed away in a shed on the South 40, start to kick in. It is like working a muscle - easy does it.

Once your body becomes keto-adapted – which may take some time based on the individual's body type, health condition, toxicity level, and determination – your body will effectively burn your stored fat. This is cool and can happen fast. There are five to six reasons the body has difficulty getting into ketosis, and we will discuss those a bit later.

**5. *What is autophagy?*** Autophagy literally translates to "eat thyself." Our bodies constantly break down old, worn-out, weak, mutating, or senescent (senile) cells. This is a self-sustaining and cleaning mechanism. The broken-down cells are then recycled for usable parts to make new cells - stem cells. Dr. Yoshinori Ohsumi won the Nobel Prize in 2016 for his work on autophagy. His discovery was, in part, that you could maximize autophagy by fasting and that by Day 3, your body was breaking down these old cells at a rapid rate. This means that we can speed up the regeneration process with fasting.

This discovery was groundbreaking in the fasting world and proved why fasting was effective.

*How does it work?* Under times of stress – in this case, the stress of not having enough food in your body – your body will look for fuel to burn inside your body in its attempt to survive. This could be likened to a bear hibernating – it's not consuming fuel; it is just burning its stored fat.

The good news is that under times of autophagy when brought on correctly, the body will look for the weakest, oldest, worn out, and mutating cells and break them down. Autophagy does not mean you are breaking down healthy cells.

Another good point is that autophagy does not just break down human cells; it also breaks down the weaker and invading microbiomes.

Autophagy allows the old cells to die and new Stem Cells to be born.

**6. *Apoptosis***. This is programmed cell death. Our cells all have a life expectancy. Once they reach the point of no return, they are programmed to self-destruct.

**7. *What are Stem Cells?*** Stem Cells are the rudimentary cells in our body. In fact, when an egg and a sperm come together, that creates a Stem Cell. That one cell then divides, replicates, and differentiates into every type of cell necessary to make a body. A stem cell can turn into over 200 different cell types based on innate intelligence and the area of the body it is working to heal.

**8. *Forever Chemicals*** - example – PFSA - Perfluoro sulfonic Acid – POPs -Persistent Organic Pollutants- which won't break down in the environment. They are a class of about 10,000 chemicals with non-stick and detergent properties now found in our waterways and soil. Of course, these PFSAs and POP chemicals have been associated with everything from cancer and thyroid disease to kidney disease and autoimmune disease.

**9. *Hormesis*** - is a characteristic of many biological processes, namely a biphasic or triphasic response to

Valter Longo, a scientist at USC, discovered (at about the same time as Dr. Ohsumi) research that stem cell production – your own body's ability to create new stem cells – was dramatically enhanced by fasting. In fact, his research indicated that stem cell production is at its highest during a five-day fast. After Day 3, the stem cells top out and stay in high production for several days.

*10. Autoimmune* – Autoimmune means your body is attacking itself. An *autoimmune* disease is when your body attacks itself, mistaking it for an invading foreign body. The immune system's job is to protect the body from invading bacteria and viruses. If the immune system mistakes your body for a foreign invader, it attacks you! Some autoimmune diseases only target a single organ, as in Type 1 Diabetes, which damages the pancreas. Different diseases, such as systemic lupus erythematosus (SLE), may affect the whole body.

*11. What are telomeres?* Telomeres are little protein strands located at the end of your chromosomes. Telomeres get shorter each time a cell divides. Eventually, the telomeres get too short and can no longer do their job, and the cells can no longer duplicate. This causes the cell to stop functioning. They act as an aging clock. These cells can mutate, become sick, or just take up space. They are dangerous, and our body should eliminate them.

But the cool thing discovered about fasting and the ketogenic diet is that, done correctly, this process can actually lengthen your telomeres, thus reversing your biological clock.

This, along with detoxifying your body of things like heavy metals, mold, and hidden infections, takes a huge load off of your body and reverses chronic disease processes by decreasing chronic inflammation.

It's like getting a new lease on life.

**12. *What is diet variation?*** Diet variation plays a big part in understanding the art of fasting. We have to go back to the early days of man - the hunters and gatherers. They based their meals on what was available and what they could hunt or gather. They didn't have a grocery store loaded with every type of food 24/ 7/ 365. They ate what was available if it was available.

First, they chased down a mammoth, then feasted on mammoth meat as their predominate food. They rendered the fat and kept it for winter, along with the nuts and roots they found. Then, often when spring came, the land was barren with little food stuffs available. This has been known as Starvation Spring. Once summer hit, there was plenty of variation and game to eat.

This gives us an understanding of diet variation. What was remarkable for these guys was that the body was constantly cleaning the house, eliminating weak cells and useless or trouble-causing microbiomes.

So, by adding diet variation into the mix, we can help the body become more efficient and healthier. In ancient times, the variation came with the season simply based on what food was available. Today, we can intersperse diet variation into our health regimen to improve our body's health. We will employ diet variation throughout our fasting. In fact, feast days (three meals a day) and famine days (twenty-four-hour fasts) are a type of diet variation.

In the bigger picture, once you reach your health goals, you may be completely out of ketosis and on a different diet for some time.

**13. What are ancient healing strategies?** Ancient healing strategies are the undertaking of the understanding we have of feast and famine and the different food types available. This way, we can challenge the body so that it is more able to handle the stresses (physical, chemical, and mental) it is confronted with.

Only the strong survive. By getting our bodies into good shape and removing toxins, such as molds, heavy metals, and hidden infections, we can boost our immune system, increase organ function, restore brain and endocrine function, and thus be ready for any flu, virus, bacteria, or other stressors we may be hit with.

***14. Metabolic Flexibility.*** As we teach our body to alternate between two fuels easily, we become metabolically flexible. This is a desirous state because it means that your body is not stuck as a glucose burner anymore and can and will use up your stored fat fuel easily, converting to a keto-burning engine on a dime to sustain energy and health. It also means that your brain is enjoying the benefits of having ketones to burn, which it loves. Another huge advantage is that you are not constantly burning inflammatory fuels like glucose to keep your body choking.

Being metabolically flexible also implies that you are not addicted to the idea that you must eat three to six meals a day, as with Western medical thinking. Instead, you are more likely to eat one to two meals a day with a feast day thrown in once a week to keep your body metabolically flexible.

Many people become part of the OMD club, meaning they predominantly consume one meal a day.

I think about this as if I were a wild animal. You don't see fat wild animals; they mostly eat as necessary to keep the body as healthy and fit as possible. The deer has to outrun the lion, and the lion must outrun the deer. Neither can afford to be overweight or in ill health.

When you think about some ancient cultures, like the great Pima Indians of the American Southwest or even some of the remote tribes in Africa today, they had/ have a diet based on what is available. They only eat what they can hunt, grow or gather. Their bodies were/ are strong, and they had/ have a strong immune system. For the Pimas, as with most all-American indigenous people, sugar, alcohol, and processed food are what did them in. As long as the tribes of Africa stay wild – the few that are – they will continue to thrive as a people.

Thus, becoming metabolically flexible is our goal.

***15. What is optimum health in this model?*** This would imply the reduction in exposure to the three major causes of stress to ourselves and our body and the correction or normalization of the population of our microbiome.

This would also include our genes' correct function and expression, meaning that our DNA is expressed optimally.

Once we determine the damage done generally and to the specific organs and systems in our body and correct them as much as possible, we can maintain this state of optimum health.

### *16. The Five Rs: The Road Map to Optimum Health*

The five Rs show us a map guiding us to better health.

***17. Remember the story of King Sisyphus?*** He was the king of Corinth in Greek Lore. His excessively proud or self-confident belief that his shrewdness exceeded that of Hades, Zeus' brother and god of the underworld, made him push a giant boulder endlessly up a hill. Once it rolled all the way down, Sisyphus would have to push it back up again.

Western medicine can be likened to Sisyphus today. Although we have the best emergency health system in the world, our "sickness care'" system is only designed to chase and mitigate symptoms until the day we die. Thus, growing old in this country can resemble a miserably pain-ful state of existence. Constantly taking a drug to cover up another symptom, suffering yet until we die – Sisyphus in the modern world.

**The Five Rs**

- **Removing** the Sources of Toxic Exposures
- **Repairing and Regenerating** the Cell Membrane (This includes repairing damage done to the gut or digestive system cell walls)
- **Restoring** Cellular Energy
- **Reducing** Inflammation
- **Reestablishing** something called methylation, proper detox pathway function, and healthy gene expression.
  - Turn on good genes
  - Turn off bad genes
  - Detoxing cells
  - Getting rid of toxic hormones

# Epilogue

I hope you found this a fun and informative way of learning about your health. The journey to better health can be a rocky road at times, but it is good to know there is a road.

I traveled this road myself. Breaking my back in that fall from a tree at age twelve set me up for a journey down a painful, drug-ridden path for the first many years of my life. It was a path full of years of self-medicating with anything from pharmaceuticals to street drugs and alcohol. It nearly killed me. I am so thankful for the two friends who carried me into Dr. Duncan McCollum's office almost forty-five years ago. If not for them, I probably would not be here today. Sadly, I don't even remember their names, but they saved my life.

The information in this book is a part of what is available to you. Each individual will have their own unique circumstances, which can require reaching deep into my bag of tricks. Oftentimes, during a detox, different situations come up. For instance, viruses, bacteria, parasites, conditions like Lyme disease, mold, and more can show their ugly head. Fear not, though. I can help with these conditions.

The path is paved. All you have to do is get on the path and let me lead you through, teaching you how to take your life back by taking your health back. You can do this!

By the way, I work with patients both in the office and virtually. I included references and links to many of the sites you will need to study if you decide to embark on this journey.

Some of you will get through the book and find it exciting but may not relate to it or believe it is something you believe is possible or for you. Thank you for your thoughts. I respect you for your decision.

Others will find it interesting and go about it themselves, learning and studying as they can. Very well – please feel free to look into all the links I provided. You are welcome to follow me at any of the below links. There are groups you can join where we have free information and even group challenges that you can participate in.

I look forward to getting to know you.

There are a lot of people who like to learn as they go and may not have the time or the urgency to delve into this as fully as others.

Then, there are those of you who need and want help now! This is where I come in. I can help you!

How to find me:

Dr. Duncan McCollum D.C. 3555 Clares St. Ste WW., Capitola, CA. 95010

(831) 459 9990

www.DrDuncanMcCollum.com

www.McCollumWellness.com

Info@McCollumWellness.com

YouTube channel: Dr Duncan McCollum

McCollumWellnessRadio@KSCO.com

Podcast: McCollumWellnessRadio

Facebook: Dr Duncan McCollum

Please join Facebook private group: Health Rebels

Instagram: @mccollumfamilychiropractic

You can find all the menus, shopping lists, worksheets, and much more at www.mccollumwellness.com

The Cellular Healing Lifestyle seven-week course can be found at McCollumWellness.com.

*McCollum Wellness*

*7-week Plan*

*YouTube Channel*

Join the McCollum Wellness Academy for ongoing support and classes.

Your first step is to go online at www.mccollumwellness.com, download and fill out the Neuro Toxic Questionnaire, and send it in. Mention that you read this book, and I will offer you a complimentary consultation to review your test results and see if any part of this program is right for you.

If I think I can help you, I will make any next-step recommendations, which may include testing or further evaluation.

I promise you this: I will help you. I will either offer you what I can to help or, if I don't believe I can help you, I will refer you to a more appropriate healthcare practitioner based on your condition.

Please note that the information in this book is given as suggestions to help you understand how to get your health back or just stay healthy. I have no intention of treating any kind of disease or health condition and recommend that you always pass any information past your medical doctor before attempting any lifestyle change, be it information in this book or information found on the internet or elsewhere.

Did you know that most people won't act? They will sit back and wonder what's happening. The magic number is 3%. History and statistics show that 3% of the people will act on any situation; the other 97% sit and wait to see what happens. I encourage you not to be in the 97%. Just look at the health statistics in our country. You can do something about it.

However, whether you decide to do nothing, peruse this on your own, or reach out so that I can help you, you have my respect and gratitude.

If you can do me one favor, please, if you know anybody who you think could benefit from this book, please
get it in their hands. It could make all the difference in the
world to them.

Much Love,

Dr. Duncan McCollum, Chiropractor

# Acknowledgments

Dr. Dan Pompa, for all the love he puts into helping others.

All my friends at Cellular Solutions, whose constant support is invaluable.

Dr. Jon Baker, for his unrelenting effort in helping me overcome my own boundaries.

Dr. Curtis Martin, for his guidance and belief in me and my dreams.

Dr. Russ Rosen, for helping me to think outside the box.

My loving family, for all the support they have given me throughout the years.

My wonderful staff, who support me in all my crazy ideas.

My amazing patients, who constantly allow me to help them with their lives.

My dad, who never lost faith in me.

My sister Sudi, who pulled me up when I most needed it.

# About the Author

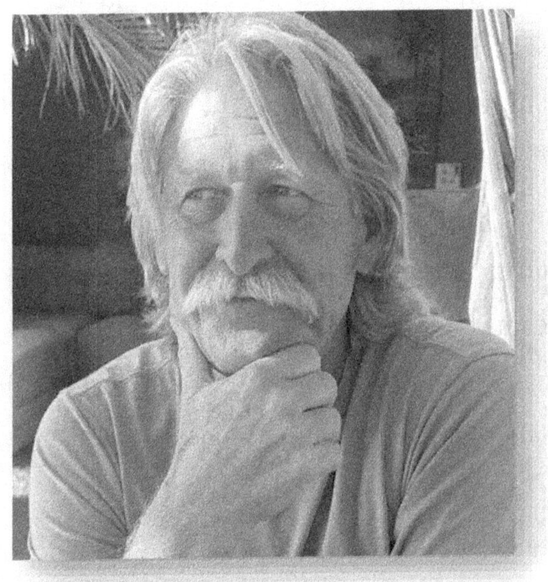

Dr. Duncan McCollum graduated from Palmer College of Chiropractic-West in 1989. He opened his practice that same year and loves serving the Santa Cruz community and, now, through the internet, the world. With a strong

interest in regenerative health, he continually strives to improve his knowledge of current natural health trends. Dr.
McCollum is a sought-after speaker, radio talk show host,
best-selling author, and, for several years, a regenerative
and cellular healing teacher.

Three principles in natural healing compel Dr.
McCollum to stay on the cutting edge of emerging health
science. Those principles are Dr. BJ Palmer's premise that
the body has an innate or inborn ability to heal itself from
"above, down, inside out," Dr. Reggie Gold's thought that
"the body needs no help, it just needs no interference," and
Dr. Dan Pompa's statement of "fix the cell to get well." As
an early adopter of cellular healing, Dr. McCollum finds
himself closely aligned with Dr. Dan Pompa, the world
leader in cellular healing. Dr. McCollum teaches the Cellular Healing Lifestyle and has become an expert in the art
of cellular detoxification. By combining these principles
with his thirty years in the chiropractic field, he has developed remarkable protocols that yield outstanding results.

Dr. McCollum understands that the way to a healthy
body is through understanding, and he lives by and loves

the old adage, "Give a man a fish, and you feed him for a day. Teach a man to fish, and you feed him for a lifetime."

# Other Books by Duncan McCollum

## Non-Fiction:

*New Hope for Sciatica: End Your Pain Now with Solutions Even Your Doctor Won't Tell You About*

## Historical Fiction:

*The Adventures of Little Big Jim*

*Coaling Station A*

*Journey's End*

*Kaleidoscope: A Glass Worth Looking Through*

www.ingramcontent.com/pod-product-compliance
Lightning Source LLC
Chambersburg PA
CBHW061620250726
48659CB00004B/1024